Praise for Teenage Anxiety

"In a time when teenage anxiety has reached unprecedented levels, Sophia Vale Galano offers something truly invaluable: a book that doesn't just explain the problem, it shows parents exactly how to help. *Calming Teenage Anxiety* isn't another guide telling parents what they're doing wrong; it's a compassionate roadmap that transforms overwhelming challenges into actionable steps. Every parent watching their teen struggle needs this essential guide."

—Kathe Crawford, master life coach and author of *Unlocking Secrets My Journey To An Open Heart*

"Sophia masterfully evokes a sense of confidence in the reader as she coaches caretakers to not only better parent their teens but themselves in the process. *Calming Teenage Anxiety* develops insight into the complex pressures adolescents experience and centers itself on the transformative role a mindful caretaker can make in a teen's life."

—Brittany Plut, LCSW, LA Integrative Therapy

"Sophia Vale Galano is the go-to expert for helping teens and their families navigate anxiety in today's world."

—Jaime Ryan, Educational Learning Specialist

"Deeply helpful, insightful, sane, grounding, sound, compassionate, informative, clear, cogent, and sensitive, *Calming Teenage Anxiety* is of tremendous value for helping parents and their teenagers in the world today. Ms. Galano is literally a lifesaver, and her expertise is a treasure."

—Phil Zuckerman, Ph.D., author of *What It Means to be Moral*

"Sophia Galano provides encouragement and a safe emotional space to engage in a much-needed conversation. As a long-time school administrator, I can think of no better resource than the guidance of a caring professional endeavoring to help teens prosper in a complex world."

—Dr. Sheril Antonio, Senior Associate Dean, Strategic Initiatives, Tisch School of the Arts, NYU

"A must-read for every parent. *Calming Teenage Anxiety* is timely, compassionate, and practical. With clarity and warmth, Sophia demystifies teenage anxiety, offers strategies that truly work, and empowers parents to gain self-awareness, empathy and understanding in order to best help their teen."

—Martha B. Koo, MD, FASAM, LFAPA, FCTMSS

Calming Teenage Anxiety

Calming Teenage Anxiety

A Parent's Guide to Helping Your Teenager Cope with Worry

Sophia Vale Galano, LCSW

Hatherleigh Press, Ltd.
62545 State Highway 10
Hobart, NY 13788, USA
hatherleighpress.com

Calming Teenage Anxiety

Text Copyright © 2025 Sophia Vale Galano, LCSW

Library of Congress Cataloging-in-Publication Data is available.

ISBN: 978-1-961293-38-0

All rights reserved. No part of this book may be reproduced, stored in a retrieval system, or transmitted, in any form or by any means, electronic or otherwise, without written permission from the publisher.

Printed in the United States

The authorized representative in the EU for product safety and compliance is Catarina Astrom, Blästorpsvägen 14, 276 35 Borrby, Sweden. info@hatherleighpress.com

10 9 8 7 6 5 4 3 2 1

Contents

Introduction ... ix

Part I: Adolescent Anxiety

Chapter 1 – Recognizing Anxiety ... 3

Chapter 2 – Biological Influences ... 11

Chapter 3 – Cultural and Social Changes: "The Gen Z Effect" ... 15

Part II: How to Help Your Teenager Cope

Chapter 4 – Preventive Care ... 41

Chapter 5 – Goal Expectations and Conveyed Messages ... 63

Chapter 6 – Communication and Monitoring Judgment ... 85

Chapter 7 – Self-Worth: Boundaries Over Restrictions ... 97

Chapter 8 – Leading by Example ... 113

Part III: Additional Support

Chapter 9 – Seeking Support ... 125

Chapter 10 – Receiving Help ... 139

Chapter 11 – Tools for Support ... 159

Chapter 12 – Additional Holistic Resources ... 181

Conclusion	185
Acknowledgments	187
About the Author	189

Introduction

I knew there was a need to write this book when I began leading presentations on adolescent anxiety. Nearly a decade ago, I was working as an associate therapist specializing in adolescent mental health. At the time, I was contacted by a high school counselor, who asked me to facilitate a discussion for parents of anxious teenagers.

Previously, I had led several presentations at different high schools on topics such as substance use, vaping, and mood disorders. However, this particular discussion on teenage anxiety struck me like none other.

As soon as I entered the room, I was amazed at how many parents were seeking guidance for their teen. I had never before presented to such a packed audience. Not only were all the chairs in the room filled to capacity, but many parents stood along the walls. As I presented and later opened the space for questions, there was an immense yearning for help among these parents. Parents were open and direct about their concerns, and were eager to learn how to support their children.

Questions echoing throughout the room included:

- "What is going on?"
- "Why are our teenagers so overwhelmed and how can we intervene?"
- "What can we do to support our teens?"

Sadly, these are not uncommon questions. I continuously receive calls from concerned parents seeking a therapist for their anxious teenager. The prevalence of teen anxiety in western culture is increasing at an alarming and severe rate. Parents are at a loss on how to handle such significant anxiety levels. Although my private therapy practice is open to teens with varying concerns, the most frequent request is treatment for anxiety disorders.

Very often, I hear horror stories of teenagers battling anxiety throughout their high school years, never receiving appropriate support and care. While some of these teens are able to persevere until graduation, many crumble once enrolled in college. Although these teens can survive at home, they are unprepared and crippled with fear when faced with independence. On the contrary, other teenagers are happy to move away and attend college, yet engage in dangerous, risk-taking behaviors to alleviate their anxiety.

I state this not to exacerbate fear and worry for the many already-concerned parents reading this book. Instead, I write this book with the intent to help you in your role as a parent, guardian, or loved one. My aim is to guide you in supporting your teenagers in coping with their anxiety, reducing anxiety levels and better preparing them for the future. While many teens may not ask for help directly, they are eager to alleviate their anxious feelings. You are a central piece of this equation.

Much like the parents who attend my presentations, you are most likely wondering how to help calm your anxious teen. Please know that you have taken an amazing first step simply by reading this book. The book is divided into three sections:

Part I: Adolescent Anxiety

Part I examines how to recognize anxiety in your teenager and explores the precipitating factors.

Part II: How to Help Your Teenager Cope

Part II explains methods of support, including preventive care, communication, self-esteem and leading by example.

Part III: Additional Support

Part III offers concrete resources for you and your teenager.

As you read, be prepared for personal self-reflection. Many of the topics and questions posed may be uncomfortable for you to consider. However, introspection is necessary in supporting your teenager. When you are your best self, you can serve as an effective support figure to those around you. While this may not be what you expected, I encourage you to maintain an open mind and a positive outlook.

There are several suggested questions and exercises listed throughout this book. While you are not required to physically write your answers, you are welcome to jot down any thoughts, ideas and themes in a journal or notebook. This can help you gain a better understanding of what occurs beneath the surface. Self-reflection is not only informative but also healing for you and your teen.

In serving as your guide, I will draw examples from my clinical work with teenagers. I will share experiences from my private therapy practice and my role as a high school counselor. Additionally, I will reference my work at adolescent mental health and substance use treatment centers. While all names have been changed, the examples provided are based upon real-life case studies.

Please note, this book is not intended as a replacement for therapy, counseling, psychiatry or medical treatment. Therapy is extremely beneficial for teenagers with anxiety and can also be advantageous for you. Complex emotions can arise while reading these pages, and it is helpful to lean on a supportive

INTRODUCTION

community. Whether your support comes from a therapist, coach or counseling group, I recommend processing your feelings in a safe manner. Furthermore, I suggest sharing this book with other parents of teenagers with anxiety, and discussing ways you can support each other.

My goal for this book is to aid your teenagers in feeling more safe, calm, and secure as they navigate life changes. Moreover, I intend to alleviate your own fears when you witness your teenager struggle. I recommend that you reference segments of this book often, re-read chapters and frequently explore your own internal concerns. Whether this is the beginning or continuation of supporting your teenager with anxiety, I encourage you to embrace hope and optimism. You are on a new path in reading this book and your future self, as well as your teenager, will thank you for it.

PART I

Adolescent Anxiety

CHAPTER 1

Recognizing Anxiety

"I lived my entire adolescence with crippling anxiety and didn't even know until beginning therapy in my sophomore year of college. I thought it was normal to feel scared, panicked and physically sick all the time. No one questioned it. Not even me."

—20-YEAR-OLD CLIENT

The first step in supporting your anxious teen is to recognize anxiety and the ways in which anxiety can manifest. Many of the parents reading this book are already aware that their teenager has anxiety. Their child is clearly struggling, and they cannot ignore or deny the challenges. However, teenage anxiety can be difficult to identify, especially for those not trained in the field of mental health.

What Does Anxiety Look Like?

Particularly in adolescents, anxiety can manifest in forms that are often overlooked or disregarded.

I commonly hear the following questions from the parents of my clients:

- "How do I know if my teenager is suffering from anxiety?"
- "What are the true signs and symptoms of teenage anxiety?"

I advise you to start reflecting through mindful and non-judgmental observation of your teens.

Ask yourself the following questions:

- Are my teenager's behaviors changing?
- Is my teenager withdrawing from social or school-related activities they once enjoyed?
- Am I noticing extreme changes in grades and academic performance?
- Is my teenager expressing more worry or fear?

- Does my teenager panic about events or school?
- Is my teenager obsessing and worrying over the future?

In considering your answers, you may find other questions arise. Some of these can include:

- "Isn't it normal for my teenager to feel this way?"
- "Don't all teenagers get moody and hormonal?"
- "Being a teenager is stressful, so wouldn't it be unusual not to feel this way?"

The answer is simple, but can be frustrating for a parent to hear. *The answer is both yes and no.*

A very simple way to understand teenage anxiety is to assess how much your teenager's behavior has changed, and how often their behavior has changed. For example, it is understandable if your teenager expresses mild nervousness about an academic test or a college interview. However, if your teenager experiences a panic attack before a math exam every week, you will want to examine further. Likewise, it is natural for a teen to be apprehensive about attending a party where they might run into former friends or significant others. However, if your teenager is terrified to meet new people or go outside, it is worth exploring deeper.

Active Listening

Mindful observation of your teenager's demeanor and actions lays a crucial foundation in recognizing anxiety. Begin by carefully listening to what your teenager communicates to you. While this might sound easy, many parents struggle with active listening, and instinctually gravitate toward providing solutions and advice.

Reflect upon the following questions:

- Is my teenager verbally stating their struggles?
- What exactly is my teenager saying and what are they describing?
- What words do my teenager use?
- How does my teenager act when speaking with me?
- How often is my teenager verbalizing challenges?
- Has my teenager stopped communicating all together?

Consider if your teenager is attempting to express their feelings to you. It is of utmost importance to listen to your teen if they are verbalizing hardship and struggle. Even if their words sound dramatic or silly, pay attention to what your teenager shares.

In my private therapy practice, many young adult clients report that their anxiety was overlooked for years by their parents. When these individuals sought help as teens, their requests were disregarded and ignored. Sadly, this is very common and can occur with even the most thoughtful and caring parents. As stated earlier, anxiety can appear in many forms and is often confused with standard teenage behavior. Ask yourself, have you ever dismissed your child's behavior as a normal part of adolescent development? Have you ever labeled their actions or communications as stemming from hormones, teen angst, rebellion or defiance?

If you answered yes, please do not judge yourself. Rather, acknowledge that your teenager may be attempting to express their struggles. Keep in mind, most teenagers are not experts at communication. Teens may not convey their challenges in the most effective and concise manner.

Cultural Considerations

"My parents view mental health completely differently than me. They were raised in a different country, went to different schools and grew up in a completely different culture than I did."

–17-YEAR-OLD CLIENT

As you reflect upon your teenager's communications, be mindful of your family's cultural background. Different cultures possess varying perceptions on mental health and anxiety. Even where you live or where you were born could influence how you interpret your teenager's emotional state. As a child growing up in England in the 1990s, I never once heard the term "anxiety" used in school or by my peers. It was not until I moved to Los Angeles at age 12 that I learned about anxiety. Culture greatly impacts how we perceive mental health conditions.

Furthermore, consider your religious or spiritual views, and how they might influence your interpretation of your teenager's communications.

Ask yourself the following questions in a non-judgmental manner:

- Is expressing fear or nervousness fairly common in my family's culture?

- Could I have misinterpreted anxiety as a cultural norm?

- Is overt fear or nervousness unusual in my family's culture?

- Are we living in an area where anxiety is not commonly addressed?

- Was I born and/or raised in a different culture or geographical area than my teenager, where anxiety was treated differently?

- Could any other cultural influences cause misinterpretation in what my teenager communicates to me (i.e., education, income, ethnicity, etc.)?

These are general questions pertaining to a larger topic of culture and mental health. The above questions are certainly not the only ones you can ask yourself, and I encourage you to explore further. As a clinician, I always consider the cultural backgrounds of my clients in order to treat anxiety most effectively. Self-reflection surrounding cultural influences can be an informative and empowering tool.

Acknowledging Confusion

Your teenager might not understand the concept of anxiety or even have a name for their suffering. Your teen may be as confused as you are. This means you and your teenager are embarking upon this journey together. Your teen may have felt anxious for a long time, or anxiety could be a new feeling. Unfortunately, the lack of understanding surrounding anxiety can be frustrating for your teenager.

Many of my adult clients did not know they possessed anxiety as teenagers. While they may have had kind, considerate parents, their parents did not fully understand mental health or ways to help. If you relate to this, please know this is nothing to be ashamed of. Instead, commend yourself for now seeking to understand anxiety.

Identifying and assigning a label to anxiety can be an enormous relief for teenagers. Your empathy and understanding will also be liberating and freeing. Overall, it is important to validate your teenagers and practice compassion. I will fully explain how to open a healthy dialogue surrounding anxiety in the chapters to come.

Continued mindful observation, active listening, and self-reflection are essential tools we will utilize throughout this book. As you read, begin to incorporate these tools into your own understanding of teenage anxiety. Understanding anxiety and possessing tools to help calm it will aid your teenager throughout adolescence and into adulthood.

CHAPTER 2

Biological Influences

"My kid doesn't have anxiety. It's just teenage hormones...right?"

–Parent of a 13-year-old client

Now that you have a basic understanding of what anxiety might look like, you may be asking, "What is causing anxiety in my teenager?" Truthfully, I could write another book to address this question. Therefore, bear in mind, the information in this chapter is a condensed answer to a complex issue. As a reminder, I am not a medical doctor and research is constantly evolving. As a whole, I have included this chapter to provide *general* information surrounding biological topics that are currently under exploration. Overall, the age-old "nature versus nurture" debate still exists, and there is no single, concrete answer. Professionals are seeking to understand the causes of anxiety – including biological factors as well as cultural, societal and environmental influences. In order to support your teenager, strive to gain a basic understanding of all aspects.

As discussed in the previous chapter, it is common for parents to confuse anxiety with standard adolescent behavior. For the purpose of better understanding your teenager's anxiety, I invite you to begin thinking about yourself as an adolescent. Reflect on your middle and high school experience. Be patient and compassionate with yourself in this reflection. I'm sure many of you would prefer to never go back to this time, even in your imagination!

Hormones, Chemical Changes and Genetics

Many of the factors contributing to teenage anxiety today are ongoing, "classic" causes that you may have experienced during your own adolescence. While some of this information might not be new to you, it is still valuable to consider. Medical researchers are continuing to explore how hormones can affect an adolescent's mood, particularly in regard to anxiety and depression. Additionally, researchers are still examining the development of the adolescent brain.

There are also thoughts surrounding genetic factors contributing to anxiety. Professionals frequently assess the link between family history of mental health disorders and the individual currently diagnosed. With this in mind, take some time to reflect on your family history in a non-judgmental manner. This might help you understand any biological and genetic influences on your teen's mental state.

Consider the following questions:

- Was there anyone in my family lineage with anxiety, depression, other mental health issues or substance use disorders?

- Were there any history of mental health/substance use concerns in the family of my teenager's other parent?

- Have I personally struggled with mental health or substance use issues?

- If my teenager is adopted, is it possible to research the family history of the birth parents? Is there a history of mental health or substance use issues in the birth family?

Please note, it is not uncommon for mental health or substance use issues to go undiagnosed in family histories. There are many reasons for this, including cultural influences, social stigmas surrounding mental health, and substance use, or simply lack of knowledge at the time.

Medical Issues

The influence of medical conditions on mental health is a crucial factor that frequently goes overlooked. Very often, clients seek therapy prior to visiting their physician. Yet a physical exam is essential for addressing anxiety effectively. Why would you, as a parent, contact your teenager's general physician because of anxiety? Unless you are working in the medical field, or have studied medicine, you might not be aware of the relationship between physical and mental health.

Medical issues can cause or exacerbate teenage anxiety. In many cases, clinicians are required to rule out a medical condition prior to forming an official diagnosis. For example, untreated thyroid disorders can often lead to depression and anxiety. Certain medications, brain traumas and other physiological conditions can contribute to a change in emotional state. I advise you to consult with your teenager's physician to ensure there are no underlying medical conditions causing anxiety.

In general, it is important not to overlook the biological factors contributing to anxiety. While I will discuss the socio-cultural influences on anxiety in the coming chapter, consider the impact of biology on your teenager. If you have additional questions pertaining to this area, speak with your teenager's medical doctor.

CHAPTER 3

Cultural and Social Changes: "The Gen Z Effect"

"My parents don't understand me. They have no idea what it's like being a teenager in today's world."

—16-YEAR-OLD CLIENT

In addition to developmental and physiological changes, there are also new precipitating factors contributing to teenage anxiety. I personally call these factors "The Gen Z Effect." Unlike the biological factors listed in the previous chapter, you might not have experienced these influences during your own adolescence. As this is a new cultural concept, the impact of "The Gen Z Effect" can be challenging to grasp.

Your Own Adolescence: A Flashback

To gain a better understanding of "The Gen Z Effect," complete this four-part exercise.

Step 1: Emotional Sense of Self

Begin by reflecting upon your own adolescence. Close your eyes to lessen distractions and obtain a clear picture of yourself in the past. If it feels helpful, reference a photograph of yourself as a teenager.

Focus on any feelings of awkwardness and uncertainty you experienced during your teenage years. Consider the ways in which you were discovering your identity and emotional sense of self. Did you feel confident and comfortable with yourself at this point in time? How did you compare yourself emotionally and mentally to others?

Step 2: Physical Changes

Bring your focus to the biological changes listed in the previous chapter, and consider what you looked like physically as a teenager. Attempt to remember the shifts that occurred in your body throughout your adolescent years.

You might laugh or cry while reminiscing, but try to ask yourself the following questions:

- Did I make some questionable fashion and hair choices?
- Did I have acne, braces or other noticeable changes that were apparent on my face?
- Was I taller or shorter than my peers?
- Did I experience puberty later or earlier than my peers?
- What was my body shape like? How did I compare myself physically to others?
- How did my physical appearance make me feel?

Step 3: Socialization

Now for the really fun part! Reflect back on your social life as a teenager. Try to remember your adolescent friendships and dating experiences.

Consider the following questions:

- Did I experience any painful rejections, judgments or early relationship breakups?
- Was I caught up in gossip and drama?
- Did I have any early sexual experiences at this time?

- How did I compare myself socially to others?
- How did my social life make me feel?

Step 4: Current Day

Perhaps you are happy, embarrassed, sad or frustrated while thinking about your adolescence. Although it can be uncomfortable, hold onto those feelings as you bring them into the current day. Imagine your experiences as a teenager, but envision these moments splashed across social media.

Examine how social media would have made you feel as a teenager. How could social media have affected your self-esteem? Moreover, how do you feel now as an adult, thinking about this? Reflect upon this and consider your teenager's relationship with social media as we continue to explore "The Gen Z Effect."

The Comparison Trap and Social Media

"Everyone's life looks so much better than mine because of what they post. It makes me hate myself even more than I already do."

—15-YEAR-OLD CLIENT

When I ask parents to partake in the above exercise, I am met with similar reactions.

Most responses are:

- "That sounds awful and embarrassing."
- "I would have hated social media."
- "I can't even imagine and don't want to imagine what that would have been like."

Even as an adult, you might find yourself caught in a comparison trap. This can occur when you read magazines, watch television and movies, work out at the gym, or pass billboards on the road. When you compare yourself and your life to others, you are caught in a comparison trap. If this is the case, do not judge yourself. Western culture conditions humans to compare themselves to others. To better understand your teenager's comparison trap, remember your teenager might be experiencing similar feelings to you. However, in addition to comparing themselves to strangers in the mainstream media, they also measure themselves against others on social media.

Social media is a tricky topic that results in confusion for many parents. This is understandable as most parents of teens did not grow up with the internet, let alone an endless number of social media platforms. Prior to the early 2000s, there were few ways to document your teenage years for the general public to assess and judge. The tendency to compare your teenage self to others mainly occurred through school, social engagements and the mainstream media. Prior to the internet, teens may have compared themselves to others while watching MTV, seeing advertisements at the mall or flipping through a magazine.

Before social media, judgments from peers would have occurred in the privacy of one's home. Even if your own adolescence was an absolute nightmare, you might have been able to escape the comparison trap at certain times of the day. Prior to social media, life outside of school could have been a time of refuge and solace.

Most teenagers today use social media as a form of social connection and communication. However, social media can create opportunities for comparison, judgment, and self-criticism. Before we move ahead, I will advise against prohibiting your teenagers from using social media. It is natural to want to protect your teens, but the approach of restriction typically backfires. Restriction can cause teenagers to feel controlled, leading to resentment and anger. Would you want to be told what to do or not to do, even if it was from a positive place? Probably not. Even as adults, we like to feel as though we can make decisions for ourselves. In the chapters to come, I will discuss how to facilitate a healthy conversation about social media with your teens. I will also share more on how to set boundaries while limiting restrictions.

Instead of prohibiting access to social media, it is better to understand the effects of social media on teenagers. In my practice, many of my teenage clients note the connection between social media and their mental health. These teenage clients also reported feeling pressured as to how they should act based on social media. Several clients expressed interest in drinking alcohol, experimenting with drugs or using nicotine due to the social media presence of individuals they look up to. It is common for teens to see others engaging in these behaviors and begin to wonder if they are "not good enough" for not partaking.

Unfortunately, I have noted a similar pattern with sexual behaviors, dating, and relationships. Many of my teenage clients have found themselves questioning their self-worth in conjunction with relationships on social media. Teenagers often link the lack of a romantic relationship with their own self-esteem. They might question, "If everyone is dating, and I'm not, what's wrong with me? Am I not good enough?" This thought process can lead to an increase in anxiety, depression or desire to act out.

Additionally, teen clients have reported feeling pressured to engage in sexual behaviors for the purpose of being seen as "good enough" and to "keep up with everyone else."

A Note on Cyberbullying

"I just don't understand cyberbullying. Thirty years ago, people would just be mean or pick on someone at school. Now it's a whole different world."

–Parent of 13-year-old client

As technology has evolved, bullying has followed in its footsteps. Social media now provides a setting for bullying, as well as a platform for self-comparison. In your own adolescence, peer-to-peer bullying was largely limited to school grounds. You were safe from bullying on weekends or afternoons alone in your bedroom. However, with the rise of social media, bullying can occur 24 hours a day, when one is in the comfort of their own home.

Cyberbullying is a serious matter that is often overlooked by parents who do not understand. Cyberbullying is a new form of harassment which most parents did not experience in their own adolescence. However, if your teenager shares that they are being cyberbullied, listen and take action. Cyberbullying can lead to many mental health concerns such as anxiety and depression.

While there are several negative aspects to social media, please know there is hope for your teenager. As a parent, you can guide your teenager in developing a strong sense of self. Anxiety dissipates when a teenager feels "good enough," has self-confidence, and develops strong self-esteem. This is an essential step to managing anxiety and will be extensively discussed in Chapter 9.

Social Media: An Ally When Used Correctly

"Social media actually made me feel safer and more confident to come out as gay."

—16-YEAR-OLD CLIENT

With a greater understanding of social media and the comparison trap, you can better understand your teenager's anxieties and the precipitating factors. However, it is equally important to examine the positive side that social media can have when used correctly.

First and foremost, social media platforms can provide fantastic resources and support for those struggling with their mental health. Many Instagram and TikTok profiles are run by qualified therapists, counselors, educators and mental health professionals. Many of these accounts list helpful coping skills and provide information surrounding positive stress outlets. In fact, many of my teenage client's report feeling more motivated and less isolated when they are following such pages.

Some social media platforms also host supportive forums and online communities for those who would like to remain anonymous in their journey of self-discovery. Several of my LGBTQ+ clients shared that social media was helpful during the process of coming out. These clients felt inspired by stories of hope and love through positive forums on social media. Additionally, social media can provide resources and support groups for those struggling with body image, sexuality, and gender identity, as well as recovery from substance use and eating disorders.

Social media can also be a platform for creativity, knowledge and charitable engagement. Creative outlets and involvement in healthy activities are wonderful ways to calm anxiety. Social media can elicit a safe space for artistic inspiration, writing, learning a new language, and involvement with a charitable cause. Overall, I have noticed a drastic shift in my clients when they began to use social media in a way that's supportive, resourceful and inspiring.

Shifting Your Teenager's Relationship with Social Media

"When I feel anxious or depressed, it helps me to go on TikTok and watch inspirational videos or check out positive pages on Instagram."

—17-YEAR-OLD CLIENT

You may be wondering how you can encourage your teenagers to change their relationship with social media from negativity and fear to positivity. Before we address communication strategies, remember that your *knowledge* about social media is helpful in itself. It is essential for you to understand how social media feeds the comparison trap when used incorrectly. Once you understand these concepts, you can have a gentle conversation with your teens about their relationship with social media.

Be non-forceful and mindful of your approach when you begin this conversation. If your teen is willing to chat about social media, place yourself in a listening and inquisitive role. Ask your teenager for their thoughts and how they feel when using certain platforms. *Listen* to your teenager without judgment or feedback. Remember, this is a starter conversation, and you do not need to provide solutions unless asked. Simply notice if your teenager is falling into a comparison trap and feeling negative. On the contrary, note if your teenager feels strengthened, accepted and empowered. If your teen is not willing to speak about this topic, respect their decision and return to the conversation at a later time.

The Highlight Reel

In asking your teenager about social media, you might receive a response such as: "I don't know. Annoyed. Bad. Sad. It's whatever. But I'm not going to stop using it. Why?"

Although you are practicing listening and observation, your teenager seeks feedback from you. Therefore, where do you go from here?

At this point, you can gently bring forth the concept of social media as a *highlight reel*. A highlight reel refers to the ways in which social media portrays only what an individual desires the world to perceive. For example, a highlight reel would not include pictures of someone watching television alone on a Friday night, waking up wearing last night's makeup, or crying over a failed test. Instead, a highlight reel would show the same person partying with friends, smiling beautifully, and succeeding at life. It is similar to how airbrushing is used in magazines and advertisements. A highlight reel is not an accurate or realistic depiction of an individual's true life.

When you explain the concept of the highlight reel, it is essential to validate your teenager's emotions. Discuss the highlight reel in an organic and conversational manner, rather than providing advice that disregards your teenager's feelings.

For example, rather than stating: "Social media is bad for you. It's just a highlight reel of someone's life and what they want to show to the world. Don't pay attention to it or let it bother you."

You could instead state: "It is completely understandable for you to feel annoyed by social media. I would be annoyed too if I saw people only post what they want others to see. It is like a highlight reel of their life. How unrealistic."

Place yourself in your teenager's frame of mind when referencing the highlight reel. Ask yourself, what would you have liked to hear at their age?

The Social Media Art Gallery

If your teenager is open to continuing this conversation, it can be helpful to explore the notion of social media as an art gallery. "The Social Media Art Gallery" places your teenager as a curator of their social media account. Unless your teenager is an artist, I do not mean encouraging your teenager to turn their account into a literal art gallery.

Rather, suggest that your teenager follow pages that elicit feelings of positivity and inspiration, as if they were curating an art gallery.

In simplest forms, curating one's art gallery might appear as follows:

- Deleting, unfollowing or blocking pages that bring forth negative emotions such as anxiety, depression and sadness.

- Following pages, accounts or people that elicit positive feelings such as inspiration, strength, empowerment and support.

- Muting or restricting people if your teenager is not ready to "unfollow" entirely. (This could eventually lead to blocking or unfollowing in the future.)

This process allows your teenager to decide what they would like in their own personal art gallery. It is crucial that you do *not* act as curator yourself, by deciding or overseeing their social media accounts. While you might be coming from a positive stance, this approach can once again backfire and cause your teenager to feel controlled. Instead, have faith in your teenager's ability to learn for themselves and trust in their process. This will be excellent for your teen's self-esteem and self-worth.

Case Study

To demonstrate the power of "The Social Media Art Gallery" I will share an example from my private practice.

14-year-old client "Lila" sought help for anxiety and depression. After a few months of therapy, Lila and I noticed she would feel a surge of anxiety or low self-worth after scrolling through social media. Lila shared she only followed her friends and influencers on social media. While she liked keeping up to date with their life events, she often found herself in the comparison trap. Lila felt "lame" and "boring" in comparison and began to judge her physical appearance.

One day, Lila shared this revelation with her mother. Lila and her mother had a positive relationship, and Lila felt comfortable speaking with her mother about anxiety and mental health. Coming from a protective stance, Lila's mother logged into Lila's account and deleted several pages without permission. Lila's mother did not ban Lila from social media, but instead decided to monitor who and what Lila follows.

Unfortunately, this caused Lila to resent her mother and feel controlled. Lila hated being treated like a child, and stopping sharing personal information with her mother.

However, after a few family sessions we were able to work out a compromise. I explained the concept of

"The Social Media Art Gallery" to both Lila and her mother. Lila's mother agreed to let Lila choose who to follow, while encouraging Lila to be mindful of the effect on her mental health. On her own accord, Lila edited who she followed by using the "restrict," "mute" and "block" settings when needed. Additionally, Lila was receptive to following supportive and inspirational pages. In doing so, Lila felt independent and respected by her mother, and appreciated being treated as a young adult, rather than a child.

Academic Competition and The Gen Z Effect

> "Whatever I do, I never feel it's enough. I need to be doing more schoolwork, taking more AP classes and leading more clubs. There is so much pressure, and I can't take it."
>
> **–17-YEAR-OLD CLIENT**

As each year goes by, I notice increased stress related to academics in my teenage clients. High schoolers are inspired and motivated to apply to colleges across the globe. While this is wonderful, with more college applications comes higher competition for college acceptance.

In addition to an increased number of college applicants, we are witnessing changes to the college application process. For example, many universities are removing the standardized testing requirement for admission. Personally, I feel this is a positive and much needed change. I am an advocate for colleges accepting students based on their individualism, rather than a numbered test score. However, in removing testing, pressure can be raised in other areas, such as academics and extracurricular activities. A high-test score could have heightened the chances of acceptance for an applicant lacking extracurricular activities. Many teenagers are unable to engage in after-school pursuits such as clubs or volunteerism due to time or financial constraints. These teenagers could have been leaning on their test-taking skills to grant them admission into college.

Whether you are for or against changes in the college admissions process, remember the impact this could have on your teenager. With enhanced competition and more change comes an increased pressure to excel academically, and to enroll in advanced or honors classes. Academic rigor requires significant coursework and study time outside of school hours. Your teenager might also feel pressured to engage in more extracurricular activities and obtain unpaid internships in order to be accepted into college. If your teen would like extra money, and finances are tight, they might also need to fit a part-time job into their already busy schedules.

You as a Teenager

To better understand this stress level, consider a typical day as a teenager in today's world.

Imagine yourself as a teen, partaking in the following activities throughout one day:

- Spending eight to nine hours in school, where you take tests, participate in class discussions, engage in group projects and have social interactions with numerous people.

- Partake in an extracurricular activity or a competitive sport requiring physical exertion.

- Working an after school job where you might be standing or moving for several hours, dealing with customers.

- Coming home, completing more schoolwork and working on college applications.

- Having dinner, showering, scrolling through social media, and going to bed.

How do you feel after thinking about this situation? I'm not sure about you, but I personally feel exhausted considering a day like this. Unfortunately, this is a typical schedule for many of my teenage clients. Moreover, it is a miracle that these teenagers manage to squeeze in an hour of therapy once a week. While we, as adults, have many responsibilities, we are fortunate that our work can (hopefully!) remain at the office, and our home can be a place of relaxation.

Mindfulness Surrounding Academic Competition

> "My parents have always overloaded my schedule with sports, clubs and activities. It's been this way since I was little. I'm worried now that if I scale back they will be disappointed. I would rather just deal with being anxious than disappoint them or have them be mad at me."
>
> **–16-YEAR-OLD CLIENT**

Be compassionate and considerate of your teenager's academic stress. This is not to suggest un-enrolling your teenager from school, telling them not to apply to college, or removing them from extracurriculars. In fact, many after-school activities can be valuable in calming anxiety. Exercise causes the body to release endorphins, creativity is a fantastic emotional outlet, and an internship or job can lead to a sense of independence and fulfillment. However, it is essential that these activities are *balanced* and not overloaded into your teenager's already busy schedule.

Reinforce your teenager's engagement in activities for enjoyment and pleasure, rather than for the purpose of achieving success. It can be harmful for teenagers to feel they need to accomplish success in order to be perceived as "good enough" or "accepted." In my therapy practice, I frequently treat teenagers who are overwhelmed with academics, internships, extracurricular activities and jobs. Many of these teens report feeling forced into these activities by their parents. While parents want their teenager to succeed, the intense drive for accomplishment can both cause and amplify anxiety.

Moreover, I often work with teenagers who are enrolled in a plethora of activities as a means of being "fixed." While activities can be beneficial for a teenager when integrated correctly, parents can take this concept to an extreme level. A parent might think, "If my child has so many outlets, activities, sports and classes, they won't have time to be anxious! They won't be sitting around dwelling on their thoughts, and if they do get anxious, they can channel it on the sports field, the dance studio, etc." This mentality makes sense in theory, but typically rebounds and causes additional stress for the teenager. Consider how you feel when you are overloaded with scheduled events and do not have time to relax. It is essential to be mindful of your teenager's schedule, stress level and how activities could impact their mental health.

Case Study

17-year-old client "Jenna" came to therapy seeking help for extreme anxiety. Jenna's anxiety was so severe that she rarely slept through the night. Additionally, Jenna constantly experienced racing, fear-based thoughts about not being good enough.

After ruling out any physical issues with her medical doctor, Jenna and I explored her daily routine and feelings surrounding pressure and stress. Jenna was a competitive gymnast, and had not taken a true day off to relax since she began high school. Jenna's weekdays consisted of attending school and then training for gymnastics for several hours in the evening. On weekends, Jenna would compete or train for an upcoming event. Even on family vacations or trips, Jenna would train in the gym for several hours.

Over time, we began to notice how school and gymnastics correlated with Jenna's anxiety. Jenna felt incredibly overwhelmed with her school schedule, training, and competitions. Jenna's parents originally suggested gymnastics as a stress-relieving exercise and a way for Jenna to fill her time constructively. Jenna's parents were supportive and encouraging of Jenna's gymnastics, and frequently registered her for more training and competitions. However, what was once a stress-relieving outlet had become the source of Jenna's anxiety.

After several months of therapy, Jenna and I explored the idea of shifting her relationship with gymnastics. Jenna worried about disappointing her parents, who had spent time and money on gymnastics. Jenna feared her parents would be angry or let down by her decision. With therapeutic guidance, Jenna was able to confront her fears in communicating these feelings to her parents. Through family sessions, Jenna's parents understood the importance of Jenna's decision making, and respected her choice to eventually leave gymnastics. Jenna's anxiety significantly decreased when she experienced more balance in her daily life.

Academic Competition and Time Off

Lastly, it is important to note the ways in which academic stress affects your teenager's free time. In my therapy practice, I am fascinated by how many teenagers feel they need to use their time off in a productive manner. A perfect example is the notion of summer vacation. Ideally, summer break is a time to regroup and prepare for the academic school year ahead.

For the teenage generation today, free time is often not truly time off. With stress and competition surrounding college acceptance, there might not be time for a relaxing and restorative summer experience. Summer vacation has become a period in which teenagers increase their extracurricular activities, seek multiple internships or enroll in college level classes. While structure and routine is valuable, many teenagers are flooded with activities. What was once a much-needed time to regroup is now a time of additional stress.

While this might sound strange, many of my teenage clients struggle to take time off to rest and unwind. With further exploration, many of these clients have also reported feeling anxious or scared they would disappoint their parents or not be accepted into college if they were to take time off. While this is alarming, anxiety surrounding time off can be prevented with your help as a parent. In the following chapters, we will examine how your teenager can achieve a healthy life balance.

A Final Note on Precipitating Factors

As we move forward in discussing how to support your teenager, remind yourself of the precipitating factors noted in this chapter. In fact, you might want to re-read this chapter a few times to fully grasp these social and cultural influences. If you have ever dismissed your teenager's anxiety as "teen angst" or brushed it aside, please do not blame yourself. Instead, continue to learn and gain new insight. Your awareness is an essential tool in building understanding and empathy for your teenager. You are already helping your teen by acquiring knowledge, and are on the right track.

PART II

How to Help Your Teenager Cope

CHAPTER 4

Preventive Care

"It's so obvious my parents have no idea how to help me."

−15-YEAR-OLD CLIENT

Part II of this book focuses on specific methods to assist your teenager in positively coping with anxiety. This chapter, *Preventive Care*, introduces four techniques to prevent anxiety in your teenager. Preventive care, often disregarded, is crucial for teenagers. Envision preventive care for mental health as you would for physical health. Just as preventive measures such as nutrition and exercise can lead to a strong physical body, preventive mental-health care can establish a healthy and anxiety-free mind.

Step 1: Initiating Conversations

First and foremost, initiate a conversation with your teenager. You might laugh and state, "I've already tried talking a thousand times. What is talking about anxiety going to do?" However, if Step 1 has not yet worked, try a new approach.

Most parents have tried to alleviate their teenager's anxiety through talking. Sadly, many go in blindly without an instruction manual. The result has been frustration and failure for both the teenager and the parents. On the contrary, a positive initial conversation can inform and validate your teenager's feelings. Validation is not only healing for your teenager but also empowering. However, it is essential this conversation is conducted in a manner that is gentle, approachable and most importantly, *relatable* to your teenager.

How *Not* to Initiate a Conversation

> "My parents tried to talk to me about anxiety by sending me a news article with statistics and graphs. It just made me feel annoyed and not want to talk to them."
>
> **–14-YEAR-OLD CLIENT**

Parents often feel they are coming from a positive place in opening a conversation, but wind up pushing their teenager even further away. Often these parents are completely confused as to what they did wrong. Prior to discussing how to initiate a dialogue, it is imperative to learn how *not* to start a conversation about anxiety.

Most importantly, an initial conversation cannot be led in an authoritative or intimidating manner. The goal of this conversation is for your teenager to feel non-judgement, care, and receptivity. Your teen seeks to feel supported, rather than fearful or judged. Therefore, if you are not in a receptive state and are unable to facilitate a non-authoritative conversation, it is okay. Simply pause and hold off on facilitating the conversation until you are open and willing to listen.

Do not begin this conversation when you have time limits, distractions or your own stresses. If you know you need to make a call in ten minutes, wait until after to speak with your teenager. If you suspect your other children will interrupt the conversation, wait until you and your teenager have privacy. If you predict the conversation will be short, still allow enough time to process. Even if your teen does not verbalize appreciation, this gesture shows respect and consideration.

Lastly, avoid bombarding your teenager with scientific definitions and statistics about anxiety. This technique rarely results in success and instead causes more annoyance in your teenager. Furthermore, refrain from referencing a textbook or reading an article in an academic manner. While your message might be accurate and well-intentioned, most teenagers already have hours of schoolwork, and do not respond well to an additional teacher-figure.

How to Initiate a Conversation

> "When I was in middle school, my friend told me they had anxiety. They said they would get scared all the time over nothing and be worried about situations that made no sense. They said their stomach would hurt all the time, and sometimes they felt they could not breathe. When my friend told me this, I felt so seen. I felt the same way as my friend. I had no idea this was anxiety and that there was a word for it."
>
> **–16-YEAR-OLD CLIENT**

In understanding how *not* to initiate a conversation with your teenager, you might ask, "How do I open a healthy line of communication?"

To begin, strive to open a dialogue that is *two-sided, respectful and considerate.* Remember, many teenagers do not know how to label the symptoms of anxiety or even verbalize the feelings. If your teenager is receptive to a conversation, and relates to this concept, validate their feelings, and mindfully explain how anxiety might look or feel.

In creating a two-sided dialogue, ask your teenager *gentle* questions. Rather than yes or no questions, ask open-ended questions about feelings related to anxiety. Specifically, ask your teenager what it feels like when they are overwhelmed, nervous or fearful. Emphasize curiosity and compassion in your questions, rather than demands and assertiveness.

Some examples of gentle questions include:

- "What are some ways you cope with stress?"
- "How do you keep calm in intense situations?"
- "What does it feel like when you have a lot on your plate and how do you get through it?"

These questions leave space for a response from your teenager. Furthermore, these questions do not include the word "*why.*" It can be challenging to not ask "why," but remember this conversation is meant to open an initial dialogue, rather than to seek solutions.

An initial conversation is not the time to seek an explanation for your teenager's stress, unless they openly share information on their own accord. If your teenager discloses the reasons they are anxious, respond by asking more open-ended questions. Once your teenager has willingly answered some of these questions, listen to their responses, and leave space for elaboration.

Listening

"My parents never listen to what I say. They just cut me off, tell me to brush it off or give me advice that I never even asked for."

—17-YEAR-OLD CLIENT

An initial conversation is a fantastic time to practice your listening skills. By listening, you might find that your teenager responds better and will be more likely to engage further. If this is a challenging concept, you are not alone. Most parents seek to fix the presenting problem and provide an immediate solution. Unless you are a trained therapist, listening can feel like you are doing nothing to help.

If listening is not your first inclination, experiment by simply nodding your head, or asking some follow up questions, such as:

- "Thank you for telling me that. Would you tell me a little more?"

- "I appreciate you sharing this with me. How often does this happen?"
- "How long have you been feeling this way and what has that been like for you?"

Listening and asking follow-up questions can be difficult at times but ultimately helps the conversation flow. Practice as much as you can and note the ways in which your teenager values your ability to listen. As a reminder, your teenager might not directly verbalize their appreciation and gratitude. However, listening is essential in providing long term support.

Clients in my private practice often share how they yearn to be listened to by their parents. Listening to your teenager shows that you value their thoughts as a young adult, rather than as a child who needs to be "fixed." As a parent, your ability to listen and engage in an inquisitive, two-sided conversation sends your teenager the message of respect. You are honoring their feelings and allowing space to share without judgment or an immediate solution. Additionally, you will earn bonus points with your teenager for treating them more like a young adult, rather than a toddler.

Again, I must stress the importance of remembering this initial conversation is for the purpose of listening only. This is not the time or place to provide solutions unless you are directly asked. Instead, this initial conversation is to open up a line of communication and create an open dialogue. You can inform and discuss anxiety with your teenager, but you do not need to "fix" everything the moment your teenager tells you they are stressed. There are some exceptions to this, such as if your teenager says they have plans to hurt themselves or others. In that case, seek immediate help by taking your teenager to the nearest hospital or calling 911.

Unless it is an emergency, remember that *listening* and opening an initial dialogue will be one of your most valuable tools. By not providing immediate solutions, you are showing your teenager it is safe to speak with you about mental health.

Step 2: Organic Discussions

Facilitating a conversation about anxiety with your teen might feel as though you are speaking an unknown language. To a certain extent, you are.

Parents often ask the following questions:

- "How do I even begin an extremely personal and intimate conversation about anxiety with my teenager?"

- "My teenager has no desire to sit down and talk with me. They would rather speak with their friends, go on social media, or basically do anything that doesn't involve talking to someone from an older generation to them! What should I do?"

Consider this secret tool: Learn to speak and understand the language of your teenager. This does not mean communicating using bizarre new slang words. Rather, speaking the language of your teenager means conversing in an *organic* manner.

You might be thinking, "That's a nice idea, but how does one form an organic conversation with a 15- or 16-year-old? I'm not even going to try." However, this is an imperative step and is accomplishable when conducted in a method that is relatable to your teen. Once again, imagine yourself as a teenager. Would you like speaking with your parents in a formalized, structured manner? Or would you prefer if conversations with your parents flowed naturally, in a more spontaneous or casual way?

Your teenager will most likely prefer the "casual, informal" option. Even in my therapy practice, it can take time for teenage clients to feel comfortable. Some teenagers begin therapy and are thrilled to let their feelings out during the first meeting. However, most require time to warm up in order to share their feelings. Some of these clients also expressed discomfort sitting in a structured environment, where we are face to face.

With these clients, I often suggest going for a walk outside, or making art while we converse. Engaging in a relaxing activity can ease discomfort and encourage more openness.

As a therapist, I found this to be a fascinating concept when I began working with teenagers. In order to facilitate an open dialogue, I placed the teenager in an environment that felt organic, natural and less structured. Due to the nature of this setting, the teenager began to feel more comfortable. I noticed the teen disclosing their feelings faster, and thus I was able to treat them more effectively.

If you already know your teenager is likely to feel uncomfortable in a formal setting, it is even more important to facilitate organic conversations and speak their language. Your teenager might have already expressed resistance toward an initial conversation about anxiety. While this can be discouraging, follow the model I use with many of my teenage therapy clients.

Informal and Less Structured Settings

Begin by creating a conversation in an alternative setting. An alternative setting can lead to less pressure in which a conversation can arise in a natural manner.

Rather than demanding your teenager sit and speak with you, instead experiment with discussions while engaging in the following:

- Driving or sitting in traffic
- Walking a pet

- Shopping
- Eating a meal together in a casual restaurant
- Sitting next to each other while having coffee, smoothies, etc.

While this can sound unusual, observe if your teenager is more open in these settings. Explore these options and think creatively about other settings for an organic conversation.

Case Study

A 14-year-old client, "Kai," came to therapy for anxiety and anger issues. During our first few sessions, Kai expressed frustration at their parents for constantly scheduling family meetings to address Kai's mental health. Kai explained how their parents would insist Kai share personal details about their life, and demanded to know what was troubling Kai. Kai felt pressured and put on the spot. Sadly, this pushed Kai farther away from their parents, who were concerned and wanted to help.

Through individual therapy sessions, Kai and I explored ways in which they could communicate this to their parents. With effective communication tools, Kai expressed their desire to discuss topics on their own terms in an organic manner. Fortunately, Kai's parents were also in therapy and discussed this concept with their own therapist. Kai's parents learned how to initiate organic conversations about mental health in a non-forceful manner.

Over time, Kai began to notice they were more receptive to conversations about mental health with their parents. In fact, Kai enjoyed talking about their personal life while driving with their parents, or after watching a television show. The informal settings allowed Kai to feel less pressured and more self-directed.

The Lives of Others

If it is still challenging for your teenager to engage in a conversation, reference examples from the lives of others. Many actors, singers and athletes are beginning to publicly share their mental health struggles. Even certain members of the British royal family are starting to embrace an openness toward mental health. As a therapist, I appreciate the ways in which celebrities break social stigmas and seek to normalize anxiety and depression. Additionally, these celebrities provide a platform in which you can begin an organic conversation with your teenager.

Engage in research surrounding these figures before speaking with your teenager. Note which celebrities your teenager likes and follows. Do an internet search on these public figures and explore their stance on mental health issues. You can then converse with your teenager about their thoughts on the celebrity's mental health struggles, supporting mental health charities, and so forth. You can gently ask your teenager if they relate, and how they feel about the celebrity's stance on mental health.

In removing the direct attention from your teenager, your teenager might be more comfortable opening up. This can sound odd to an adult, but remember, you are communicating with an adolescent, and it is crucial to speak their language.

Entertainment Time

"This sounds kind of weird, but I watched an episode of my favorite teen show with my mom. It was kind of awkward at the time, but we ended up having a whole conversation about sex and drugs afterwards. I feel like I could actually be real with her and that was really cool. I don't think we would have spoken about those things without watching that episode."

–17-YEAR-OLD CLIENT

The following concept can sound even stranger than relating to the lives of others. Regardless of whether your teenager is receptive to a discussion on anxiety, watch television shows and films together.

Mental health is a relevant topic in today's society and is frequently depicted in current media. Many television shows and films portray characters struggling with mental health concerns, including anxiety, depression, trauma and addiction. While this cannot be said for every film and television show, Hollywood is making tremendous efforts to accurately portray these issues. As a therapist, I volunteer for a non-profit called Hollywood, Health and Society at the USC Norman Lear Center. This organization recruits mental health and a range of medical professionals for expert consultations and to review scripts for accuracy in their depiction of mental health storylines and a wide range of medical topics. I have personally witnessed the great lengths filmmakers and television writers work in order to achieve accurate portrayals of mental health concerns.

Films and television shows conveying realistic mental health issues are a great way to begin an organic conversation. Engage in more research, but this time, explore contemporary television shows and films. Search options that could relate to your teenager's anxiety and also be of interest to your teen. Remember, you will be watching these films and television shows together. Most likely, your adolescent will be more interested in a current teen drama than a documentary from forty years ago. However, chat with your teenager, and ask what sounds intriguing.

Be mindful as many television shows depicting teen anxiety can be rather controversial. I frequently receive resistance from parents when I suggest watching current teen dramas, even with older teenagers. These shows can be explicit and feature disturbing content. They might also be sexually graphic and can be triggering for certain viewers. Therefore, if you do not feel comfortable watching with your teenager, I respect the decision.

In addition to anxiety, many current teen dramas address trauma, sexual assault, suicide and substance abuse. These are serious situations affecting many teenagers today and require informed conversations. Please do not avoid addressing these topics, as difficult as they might be. Just as I recommend beginning a preventive conversation about anxiety, I also advise you to preventively discuss other mental health concerns.

Overall, be selective and use your own discretion in deciding what to watch. If it assists you in your research process, you can also watch shows alone before viewing them with your teen. This way, you can better assess your comfort level and decide how you would feel watching with your teenager. I will also note, many teenagers decide to watch these shows on their own anyway. If this is the case, ask if you can join your teenager in the process, and use it as an opportunity to discuss mental health.

Lighter Entertainment

It is understandable if you do not feel comfortable watching graphic programs with your teenager. For example, if your teenager has a history of trauma or sexual assault, an explicit teen drama might not be appropriate. Some films and programs can be triggering for your teenager. However, if you like the idea of connecting with your teenager through entertainment, there are other options.

You can watch other films and television shows that are a little lighter in their execution. Not all programs about mental health are disturbing, and lighter options can still be a starting point for effective conversations. Contemporary documentaries and docu-series can also be informative and entertaining. However, please research documentaries to ensure they are current and up to date. Remember, the goal is for your teen to relate to the program and eventually share their own feelings and thoughts on mental health.

Following Up

Speaking with your teenager about their thoughts on the program is an excellent way to begin a conversation. Ask your teen how they felt about the characters and their various mental health concerns. If your teenager is receptive, you can ask what anxiety might have felt like for the characters, or what your teenager thinks could have helped. If the conversation feels positive, you can then gently relate this back to your teenager.

Most importantly, ease your teenager into a conversation about themselves, and as always, do not force your teenager to converse. If your teenager is willing, you can continue a preventive conversation about anxiety. Ask thoughtful questions in a non-intrusive manner.

Some questions might include:

- "How about you? How do you relate to these characters?"
- "What is it like for you when you feel that way?"
- "When you feel anxious, sad, or overwhelmed, how can I support you and be there for you?"

Anxiety can be shameful and scary, particularly when one does not truly understand. However, if your teenager is receptive, you can explain what anxiety might look and feel like to an individual. Reference the characters in the entertainment program, as well as your teenager's responses to the questions.

Use this follow up conversation to normalize topics surrounding mental health. By discussing mental health in an open-minded, realistic and nonjudgmental manner, you create a safe space for your teenager. In examining topics such as anxiety, you are taking another crucial step in being a resource for your teenager.

Step 3: Relating

> "I'm lucky because my dad really understands anxiety. I know he also experienced anxiety as a teenager and went to therapy. I never feel judged talking to him because I know he gets it."
>
> —14-YEAR-OLD CLIENT

Relating is a challenging concept for many parents. As with Step 2, Organic Discussions, relating might entail speaking with your teenager in an unfamiliar manner. In relating, you *mindfully* speak with your teenager more like a young adult, rather than a child.

If you struggled with anxiety during your own adolescence, disclose your experiences to your teenager. However, be mindful of *how* you disclose, *what* you disclose, and *how much* you disclose. Maintain boundaries and avoid oversharing unnecessary information. Rather, comment on the ways in which you relate, and highlight your own experiences. It can be helpful to share how you overcame your challenges in a non-forceful manner. Listed below are some examples of *unhelpful relating, vs helpful relating*:

Case #1

Unhelpful Relating

"Oh my God, I have crippling anxiety too and the world is awful, and it never gets better. Also, your brother (sister, father, mother, grandparents) makes everything worse for me and the whole world is out to get me."

Helpful Relating

"I understand how you feel. I also struggled with anxiety in the past and know what it is like to be overwhelmed. It felt really helpful and empowering for me to talk about it.

What is it like for you to talk about it?"

In the "unhelpful relating" example, the teenager is indirectly told that anxiety is permanent and there is no hope. The "unhelpful relating" example also victimizes the individual, which is the opposite message you want to portray. The goal in relating is for your teenager to perceive themselves as strong and resilient, not as a helpless victim. On the contrary, the "helpful relating" example validates the teenager's feelings, and enhances solidarity. Additionally, the "helpful relating" example encourages empowerment and offers reflective questioning.

Case #2

Unhelpful Relating

"I have the worst anxiety ever and it's just constant and doesn't stop. But you are not alone because I deal with it all the time. Let me tell you all about it, and then maybe you can tell me what to do since you are so smart and good at fixing things."

Helpful Relating

"I hear you and relate to what you are going through. I am happy to share more if you would like to hear what helped me, but only if that would feel good for you. I would also like to know how I can support you through this."

The "unhelpful relating" example is a common way parents attempt to relate to their teen. This frequently occurs in parents who are very close and connected to their teenager. These parents have positive intentions in their attempt to relate, connect and empower their teenager (i.e., "You aren't alone here," "You are so smart and good at fixing things.") However, the "unhelpful relating" example depicts conflicting roles among the parent and teenager, which can ultimately lead to an increase in anxiety. The "helpful relating" example provides a healthy balance of appropriate relating while maintaining parental roles and placing focus on the teen.

There are numerous benefits of healthy and appropriate relating. Relating to your teenager's emotions can be healing as well as a productive way to normalize feelings. Relating can allow your teenager to feel safe, validated, and less emotionally isolated. Additionally, many of my clients share that they feel safer confiding in a parent who has overcome similar hardships. These clients reported feeling less anxious when learning they are not alone in their struggles.

Relating requires mindfulness of boundaries and practicing balance. While relating might require speaking to your teenager more like a young adult, remember you are still the parent, and your teenager is still your child. Even if you and your teenager are close, you are conversing with your teenager—not your best friend, therapist or life coach.

Step 4: Keeping an Open Dialogue

Now that you have created an initial dialogue about anxiety, do not let your first conversation be the last. Check in with your teenager and maintain an open line of communication. Follow up with your teenager from time to time and ask how they have been feeling since you last spoke.

Maintaining an open dialogue does not mean creating an excessive, controlling or "helicopter" dynamic. This often occurs among concerned parents who mean well, but end up further isolating their teenager. While it can be difficult, refrain from constant questioning, check-ins, and ignoring requests for space from your teenager. If you relate to this, do not judge yourself as it is natural to want to help. Simply remember that balance is essential, and be mindful of how often you check in.

If this is a challenging concept to understand, consider how you feel when someone constantly calls you. Even if the person calling is someone you love, by the tenth time your phone rings, you might start to get annoyed. You might even begin to dread interactions with the person on the other end of the line. This is how your teenager can feel if you constantly force conversations about mental health. It is imperative to allow your teenager to still have space while maintaining an open dialogue.

Even if your initial dialogue does not turn into a lengthy conversation, do not be discouraged. You are following a positive path by starting to normalize topics surrounding anxiety. Remember, preventive care is about *beginning* a conversation with your teenager. We will discuss how to continue communication in Chapter 7, but for now, know you have initiated a highly important process. This can take time, so practice patience and self-compassion.

CHAPTER 5

Goal Expectations and Conveyed Messages

"My parents expect way too much from me. It's just not realistic and they can't accept it. They want to help me but refuse anything less than perfection."

–17-YEAR-OLD CLIENT

After reading the previous chapter, you hopefully began a preventive care conversation with your teenager. If your teenager was resistant, and the conversation did not occur, please do not give up. Moreover, if your teen is past the preventive care stage of anxiety, it is not too late. There is hope to heal and you can still support your teenager throughout their journey. This chapter will examine detailed methods to help your teenager lessen their anxiety.

As a disclaimer, it is common for personal resistance to arise while reading this chapter. The self-reflective exercises listed below can feel more intense than in the previous chapters. Therefore, take your time and be kind to yourself throughout the process. Do not overly criticize yourself as you explore goal expectations and conveyed messages.

Instead, reflect on the topics in a mindful and observant manner. Remember, no human is perfect, and it is natural to discover areas in need of improvement.

Gaining Empathy and Understanding: A Reflective Exercise

In order to begin examining goal expectations, I recommend the following reflective exercise:

> *Think of yourself today as an adult. Imagine spending every day in a job you do not like. Your boss pressures you to complete difficult assignments under short deadlines. You struggle to complete these tasks and have little interest in your work. Additionally, your co-workers are competitive,*

> and perhaps even threatened by you because of their own stress level. Your co-workers might have low self-esteem and lack a sense of self, causing them to lash out at you. You are surrounded by people experiencing their own personal challenges, and difficulties communicating their feelings. When you return home, your family pushes you to work harder, try harder and do more. You feel trapped and do not know how to change your life. Imagine living in that environment for four years.

In order to fully evaluate goal expectations and conveyed messages, it is critical to understand the lifestyle of teenagers today. How did the exercise above make you feel? Did any feelings of stress, anger, fear and/or anxiety arise? Unfortunately, the scenario described is often similar to a teenager's high school experience. Pressure from authority figures, competitive peers and demanding deadlines are common for the average teen. While you might not directly relate to your teenager in many ways, you can show support by increasing empathy.

Empathy does not mean acting drastically, such as removing your teenager from school or completing their homework yourself. However, an empathetic understanding of your teenager's stress will help you in exploring the next two concepts.

Goal Expectations

Truthfully examine the expectations you place on your teenager. To clarify, ask yourself the following questions regarding different areas of your teenager's life:

Academics

- What are my thoughts regarding my teenager's academic performance?
- What are my feelings surrounding my teenager's enrollment in AP and honors classes?
- What are my beliefs on grades and GPA?
- What is my stance on my teenager's participation in extracurricular activities, internships and after-school jobs?
- What are my expectations surrounding college acceptances?
- What is my response when my teenager makes an academic mistake?
- Are my academic goals realistic and accomplishable by a teenager in today's society?

Social

- What are my thoughts surrounding my teenager's social life?

- How do I respond when my teenager makes a social mistake (becoming friends with the wrong people, breaking up with someone, etc.)?

- Do I allow my teenager to decide for themself who they socialize with?

- Are these realistic social expectations for a teenager in today's society?

Emotional

- What is my response when my teenager shows their emotions?

- Do I ever tell my teenager how they should feel?

- Are there expectations for my teenager to feel the same as me?

- Are these approaches emotionally helpful for a teenager in today's society?

Reflect on your answers to these questions. Do your responses fall in a demanding or restrictive category? Could your answers lead to unrealistic and unsuccessful outcomes? Overall, are you expecting too much from your teenager? If you answered yes, do not blame yourself. High expectations can arise from loving parents who desire the best for their teenager. However, in order to support your teen, consider compassionately modifying your goal expectations.

Goal Modification

You might now be asking, what is goal modification and how do I modify with success? Goal modification is changing the expectations you have for your teenager. Reference the questions above and note the areas in which you can change your goal expectations. Do your best to remain empathetic and understanding of your teenager during the process. This will help you modify goals with success. Some examples might include:

Academics

- Settle for a fewer AP and honors level classes
- Accept your teenager might not earn a 4.0 GPA
- Practice compassion surrounding the college application process

Social

- Allow time for socialization
- Lessen judgment when your teenager makes a social mistake
- Do not control who your teenager chooses to date (unless illegal or would cause imminent harm)

Emotional

- Refrain from providing immediate solutions or "I told you so" statements
- Allow your teenager to express their feelings, even when you feel they are wrong
- Accept you and your teenager will feel differently at times

Modifying and changing goal expectations can be very upsetting for some parents. Parents with high expectations typically possess positive intentions and do not mean to cause harm. These parents might believe in their teenager's capability and feel their teen simply requires motivation. However, it is crucial to differentiate between helpful encouragement and unrealistic expectations. Encouragement can be empowering, whereas forceful demands can increase anxiety.

Goal Modification vs Enabling

As you practice goal modification, it is of utmost necessity to refrain from enabling your teenager. Enabling patterns are the opposite of demanding or unrealistic goal expectations. Enabling reinforces negative behavior through lack of boundaries or healthy consequences. Enabling can be difficult to identify, as it can appear more subtle, and is easily confused with caring or compassionate behavior. In modifying your goal expectations, seek to find a balance, rather than an extreme all-or-nothing approach.

The examples below illustrate the differences between unrealistic goal expectations and enabling scenarios.

Academic

Unrealistic Goal Expectation: Demanding straight As, and all honors/AP classes.

Enabling Scenario #1: Accepting all Ds and Fs. Allowing your teenager to skip school and not complete their school assignments.

Enabling Scenario #2: Your teenager struggles academically. You complete your teenager's school assignments so that they receive straight As.

Social

Unrealistic Goal Expectation: You expect your teenager to make academics and extracurricular activities their entire life. You limit socialization with friends and do not allow dating.

Enabling Scenario #1: You let your teenager skip school to spend more time with friends and email their teachers for extensions on assignments.

Enabling Scenario #2: You allow your teenager to spend time with whomever they want. You teenager starts using drugs with these friends and begins getting in trouble with authority figures. You take no action.

Emotional

Unrealistic Goal Expectation: You expect your teenager to be composed emotionally, and never express anger or sadness.

Enabling Scenario #1: You allow your teenager to scream and curse at you when they are angry.

Enabling Scenario #2: Your teenager cries to you constantly and you ignore pleas for help.

Although these examples might sound extreme, enabling is highly destructive and problematic. Examine if your goal modification, or other patterns of behavior are enabling your teenager. While we will discuss boundaries versus restriction in Chapter 9, if you are struggling with enabling behavior, consult with a mental health professional.

Conveyed Messages

Your teenager might be highly attuned to the world around them. They might possess an insightful awareness regarding people and situations. On the contrary, your teenager might appear completely checked out. Perhaps they are more absorbed in video games and social media than what is occurring right in front of them. Regardless of how your teenager appears, *they are highly observant of their parents*. However, most teenagers are not outwardly aware of their own observance. This process can occur on both a conscious and subconscious level. Meaning, your teenager is constantly noticing your words and observing your actions.

To understand the significance of your words and actions, reflect on the messages you convey to your teenager. Do not be worried if you are unsure of your answers, or if you feel conflicted and unsettled in considering your responses. This exercise is simply to start thinking about your influential power.

Ask yourself the following questions:

- What messages am I conveying to my teenager?
- How could my words affect my teenager's anxiety?
- Do my daily messages convey fear, concern or my own anxieties?
- Do I regularly speak to my teenager from a position of trust and safety?

Most parents do not realize the significance of daily interactions with their teen. Some parents understand how overall parenting style can affect their teenager's emotional development but overlook the small details. However, it is necessary to remember how small interactions with your teen can shape their impression of the world.

In order to explore your conveyed messages, it is essential to examine three factors:

1. Word choice
2. Tone of voice
3. Overall energy

Word Choice

Consider the power of spoken words. Words can be used to declare wars and incite acts of hate. On the contrary, words can express feelings of care, love and comfort. Think of the powerful statement, "I love you." Recall the first time you heard these words from a romantic partner. Do you remember the feelings? Hearing the words "I love you," can bring back intense memories and emotions.

With this in mind, consider how your word choice can affect your teenager. Reflect on the typical words and phrases you choose when you communicate. Hopefully, you do not use words and phrases that demean or belittle your teenager. You do not curse at your teenager, tell them they are less than, or intentionally hurt their feelings. Any words that fall within these categories are unacceptable when communicating with your teenager. Please remove them from your vocabulary as soon as possible.

Furthermore, there are statements that can appear harmless, but are quite charged. These phrases do not evoke sharp, overtly negative feelings, such as curse words. However, they can subtly convey unhelpful messages that create and enhance anxiety.

These statements are:

- "You have to…"
- "You need to…"
- "Why can't you…"
- "You should be…"

Reflect on how often you use these statements with your teenager, as well as other individuals in your life. Consider how you feel when someone uses these phrases with you. How does it affect you when a family member tells you how you should act or feel? How do you feel when your co-workers tell you what you need or have to do? Most people respond in a negative manner to these statements.

These phrases are frequently used by well-meaning individuals who have little clue about their negative impact. I recommend avoiding these statements with your teenager, as well as with yourself. Consider the pressure behind these phrases. How do you feel reading the following examples?

When communicating with your teenager:

- "You *have to* take more advanced placement courses."
- "You *need to* not be so angry."

- "Why *can't* you make more friends?"
- "You *should be* doing so much more."

When communicating with yourself:

- "I *have to* go on a diet."
- "I *need to* not be so miserable."
- "Why *can't* I do more with my life?"
- "I *should be* more successful."

Instead of using these phrases, I suggest conveying your message using different language and vocabulary.

Some options might include:

- "I would like you to…"
- "I feel it could be helpful to…"
- "What are your thoughts on…?" (Posed as a question)
- "It might be worth it to…"
- "I believe in you to…"

Explore how you feel when conveying similar messages with different words and phrases.

The same examples are listed below:

When communicating with your teenager:

- "*I would like you to* take more advanced placement courses."
- "*I feel it could be helpful to* not be so angry."
- "*What are your thoughts on* making more friends?"
- "*I believe in you to* do so much more."

Communicating with yourself:

- "*I would like to* go on a diet."
- "*I feel it could be helpful to* not be so miserable."
- "*What are my thoughts on* doing more with my life?"
- "*I believe in myself to* be more successful."

Overall, lean on phrases and words that elicit choice, empowerment, and resilience. Do your best to avoid statements that evoke judgment and promote feelings of shame and belittlement. If you feel confused or unsure, I advise using more "I" rather than "You" statements. Turning phrases into questions is another helpful technique, as questions can prompt further exploration and conversation. As always, there are of course emergency situations in which you will want to state "You have to" or "You need to," due to medical necessity or a matter of safety.

A Final Word on Words

Interestingly, word choice is frequently discussed in the context of romantic relationships and throughout couple's therapy. Sadly, word choice is often disregarded in parenting and treating teenage anxiety. While romantic relationships differ from parent-child relationships, word choice is equally as valuable. Moreover, words are powerful in *all relationships*, including significant others, family members, friends, co-workers and colleagues.

Most importantly, improved word choice is a subtle yet powerful tool you can employ immediately. Additionally, this requires no action from your teenager and is entirely in your control. This can be particularly relieving if a teen is resistant to help and engaging in a dialogue. Begin to experiment by carefully selecting the words you use with others, as well as with yourself. With patience and attention, you will begin to notice a positive change.

Tone

"My parents literally demand that I tell them what's going on in my life. They say it could help me, that they love me and they want me to be better. But them demanding and almost yelling at me just turns me off."

–15-YEAR OLD CLIENT

Tone of voice can sound like another small detail to overlook. You might already know it is counterproductive to yell or scream at your teenager. However, have you ever placed significant thought to your tone of voice in general? Moreover, have you considered your response to the tone of voice among other people in your life?

Consider the tone of voice typically used by people in different professions. Therapists are encouraged to speak in a slow, calm manner to help ease their clients. Lawyers often lean on clear, demonstrative and perhaps even stern speech to win a case in court. If you have ever listened to a guided meditation, you know that a frantic, fast-paced voice will not help you relax.

Very often, I work with parents who use the correct words when communicating with their teenagers but undermine the message with an ineffective tone. Their words have little impact, as their tone of voice conveys anger, impatience, judgment, or disappointment. Close your eyes and picture someone stating "I love you" while screaming angrily at their partner. This will have a very different effect than someone stating, "I love you" in a calm and kind manner.

Bringing awareness to your tone of voice can be helpful when communicating with your teen. Ask yourself if and when it would be beneficial to slow your pace and relax your tone. This is particularly useful when facilitating an initial conversation with your teenager. Stating "I would like us to have a chat," in a warm tone is more inviting than using a demanding voice. A softer, calmer tone of voice can elicit feelings of comfort and care, rather than fear and dread. While there is of course a time and place for a stern tone of voice, do not use this approach when initiating a two-sided dialogue. A negative tone of voice can create defensiveness and animosity, whereas a positive tone of voice can welcome and heal. Tone of voice is also connected to the final factor in conveyed messages, overall energy.

Overall Energy

"It's kind of weird, but I've started to notice I have the same fears as my mom. I feel like I'm anxious about the same things as her. She gets really

> anxious around big crowds. I get anxious around big crowds. My mom was always scared I was going to get kidnapped as a child. Now I'm always scared I'm going to get kidnapped, so I don't want to go out alone. I feel like she's scared about so much. I'm scared too and I really don't want to be."
>
> —13-YEAR-OLD CLIENT

How often do you consider your overall energy? Much like word choice and tone, most people live their life without a thought on how they present themselves energetically. Western culture emphasizes external presentation; how one looks and what others visually notice. However, in helping your teenager cope with anxiety, you must become mindful of your overall energy.

Ask yourself the following questions:

- How do I feel when someone around me is stressed or nervous?
- How do I feel when someone around me is angry or sad?
- Do I find myself absorbing the emotions of others (e.g., becoming stressed if the person near me is stressed, getting angry if someone close is angry)?

Some people are unaffected by the emotions of others. These individuals have no problem detaching and do not absorb the energy of those around them. There is absolutely nothing wrong with this. In fact, many individuals find this to be an easier, more peaceful way to live. However, other individuals (particularly those prone to anxiety) are highly sensitive to other people's energy and emotions. Often, teenagers with anxiety are tremendously empathetic and have difficulties *not absorbing* the energy of others.

Many parents laugh and disregard the importance of energetic awareness. It might seem too new-age, spiritual or unconventional. However, this type of energetic awareness has little to do with burning incense and chanting. Your energetic awareness is profoundly important as energy conveys messages to your teenager. This is why it is imperative to engage in self-reflection and note your own fears and anxieties.

Therefore, ask yourself:

- How do I handle stress?
- How often does my teenager see me flustered, panicked, nervous or worried?
- What message does my own anxiety send to my teenager?
- Am I fearful and concerned about the world around me?

- Have there been times when my own worry, fear, concern or panic caused my teenager to feel similar emotions?

If you answered yes to any of the questions, do not be upset with yourself. Fear, concern and worry are natural responses to the stressors of life. However, note how your teen might absorb your anxious energy, particularly if they are sensitive and empathetic. Your teenager might not even be conscious of their own empathic nature, and how they follow your energetic lead.

In bringing your awareness to your own energy, you might ask what to do next. Does this mean you need to hide all of your fearful emotions from your teen, and act relaxed when you are completely terrified? Definitely not. Your teenager will read right through your pretense. Additionally, pretending and hiding emotions teaches your teenager to also shield their feelings. Instead, seek balance by processing your own anxieties with a counselor or therapist. We will discuss this in Chapter 8, but for now, begin to recognize how your personal well-being strengthens the emotional wellness of your teenager.

CHAPTER 6

Communication and Monitoring Judgment

"Whenever I try to talk to my kid, she thinks I'm trying to pick a fight. I'm just trying to communicate."

–Parent of 14-year-old client

Open and effective communication is a pivotal tool in supporting your teenager. Even if you are far past the preventive care stage of support, reference and utilize the skills described in the previous chapters. As a reminder, lean on organic, non-forceful ways to elicit discussions and relate when appropriate. Be mindful of your words, tone and overall energy.

The Hot Topics

You might have already mastered the basics of communication with your teenager. Your teenager could be forthcoming about their mental health and feelings surrounding anxiety. However, is your communication solely limited to conversations about mental health? Or do you and your teen speak about other personal, often uncomfortable topics?

To clarify, consider how you and your teenager communicate about the following subjects.

If you have never discussed these topics, note any feelings that arise as you envision the conversation:

- Overall sense of identity
- Gender
- Sexuality
- Sexual health
- Dating and relationships
- Substance use

How did it feel to reflect on these topics? Did certain subjects feel more challenging, or elicit feelings of discomfort and uncertainty? On the contrary, which topics are you more comfortable and confident discussing with your teen? Most importantly, note what makes you feel hesitant or even scared to address.

As always, acknowledge your feelings mindfully and without judgment. It is common for parents to avoid bringing forth these topics due to fear, nervousness or lack of awareness. Many parents believe their teen is too young to discuss topics such as sexuality, gender identity, and substance use. Some parents also fear these subjects could corrupt their teenager.

While these feelings are valid, *teenagers are not too young to discuss these subject matters*. Additionally, teenagers are most likely already aware of these topics and were previously exposed to them in middle school. In the unlikely event your teenager does not already know about these topics, they will learn eventually. Do not try to protect your teenager by avoiding difficult conversations.

Facing Discomfort

Even if you dread the idea of speaking with your teenager about challenging subject matters, I urge you to face your fears. The above topics can be an immense source of anxiety for teenagers. It is critical not to avoid these topics if you truly want to support your teen.

Instead, empathize with a teenager's anxiety in experiencing the following:

- Early sexual experiences
- Questioning their sexual and/or gender identity
- Coming out to their friends and family
- Feeling pressured to experiment with drugs and alcohol
- Experiencing first love and heartbreak

Speak with your teenager about these subjects in an open and non-punitive manner. Refrain from insisting your teenager never have sex, drink alcohol or smoke marijuana. This is unrealistic and conveys the message that your teenager cannot share with you. Instead, set appropriate boundaries, and teach your teen about safe practices. For example, rather than stating "You are not allowed to have sex until college," teach your teenager about the importance of contraception. Similarly, rather than saying, "You are never allowed to have alcohol while living here," you can emphasize the importance of not drinking and driving.

The Consequence of Avoidance

Unfortunately, there can be serious consequences when parents do not discuss these topics with their teenagers. If a teenager cannot confide in or ask their parents questions, who can they turn to? Some teenagers are lucky to have older siblings, mentors, teachers or mental health professionals that can provide direction. However, most teenagers seek education on these topics through incorrect and misinformed sources.

Case Study

17-year-old "Jamie" came to therapy for anxiety and low self-esteem. After several months, Jamie disclosed his fears and anxieties surrounding sex and dating. He had little prior sexual experience and was worried about body image and performance. Jamie had never spoken with his parents about sex other than a conversation consisting of "just use a condom" when he was 15.

Jamie admitted he was confused about typical or "normal" sex. He had spoken with his friends about their sexual experiences, only to learn they were just as inexperienced and clueless. In middle school, Jamie decided that watching pornography would be a helpful way to learn about sex.

> From watching pornography, Jamie developed inaccurate ideas and unrealistic expectations. Jamie's incorrect perceptions regarding body image led to fears surrounding sexual performance. As a result, he developed extreme anxiety about sex.

Jamie's story is not an uncommon scenario. Unfortunately, the majority of teenagers today learn about sex through pornography. Similarly, teenagers learn about substance use from trying alcohol and drugs firsthand. On the contrary, when you openly discuss challenging topics with your teenager, you provide a safe platform for correct information. Your teenager might appear resistant, annoyed or embarrassed at first. However, open communication reduces stigmatization,shame and misinformation. Additionally, discussing challenging topics allows your teenager to turn to you when needed.

Monitoring Judgment

"My mom doesn't realize how judgmental she is. She has a negative opinion about most people and their decisions. That's why I don't share things with her."

–16-YEAR-OLD CLIENT

Perhaps you check all of the boxes in regard to communication. You openly speak with your teenager about everything from substance use to gender and sexuality. However, your teen is still anxious and resistant to communication. If this is the case, I encourage you to explore your personal relationship to judgment. Could your teenager be internalizing any subconscious or conscious judgments from you?

In order to assess, ask yourself the following questions:

- Am I critical or disapproving of my teenager's choices and decisions?

- Do I judge or criticize my teenager's friends or romantic interests?

- When my teenager makes a mistake, do I ever state, "I told you so?"

- Could my protective nature be misinterpreted as judgment?

It is natural if you catch yourself judging and answering yes to the above questions. You might even notice yourself judging me for asking you these questions. You might now be judging yourself for being judgmental! Judgments are often unintentional and arise from a place of protection. Some of the most judgmental parents I know are those who are highly protective of their children. These parents are often unaware how their protective nature comes across as critical and disapproving. However, when teens feel judged, they can become distant, non-communicative and anxious. Remember, teenagers seek approval from their parents, whether it is verbalized or not. In order to support an anxious teenager, it is crucial to monitor your judgment.

The Judgment Zone

Even if you rarely criticize your teenager directly, it is still beneficial to explore any deeper, underlying judgments. In particular, examine how your teen receives your judgments and disapproval of other people. Moreover, assess judgments about your personal sense of self, self-worth and self-esteem. While this is rarely purposeful, your teenager could internalize your judgements towards yourself and others.

Consider asking yourself the following questions:

- How often do I outwardly disapprove of or judge other people in my life? (i.e., co-workers, family members or friends)

- How often do I judge or criticize people who look physically different than me? (i.e., gender, race, body shape)

- What judgments do I make about people who are different from me in other ways? (i.e., socioeconomic class, income level, sexual orientation)

- Do I verbally judge myself? (i.e., appearance, body image, career success)

Reference your answers in reading the following two case studies.

Case Study #1

14-year-old "Justin" came to therapy for anxiety and depression. During our initial session, Justin stated he felt supported by his parents. Justin's parents did not criticize Justin when he made mistakes and instead encouraged learning from experience. Justin's parents rarely judged his academic or extracurricular choices and allowed Justin to make his own decisions.

After a few months of therapy, Justin disclosed he was confused about his sexuality. About a year ago, Justin noticed he was developing romantic feelings for his male best friend. This was also when Justin noticed the onset of his anxiety and depression.

While Justin felt supported by his parents in most areas of life, Justin knew his father was uncomfortable around gay males. Although never directed at Justin, Justin's father would often state homophobic comments in passing. While non-intentional, these comments negatively impacted Justin's mental health. Justin internalized these judgments and became fearful his father would not approve of Justin's sexuality.

Fortunately, Justin was eventually able to come out to his parents. With the help of therapy, Justin communicated his feelings about judgments to his father. Justin shared how these comments hurt his feelings and increased his anxiety and depression. With encouragement, Justin's father learned to stop verbalizing judgments about homosexual men. While Justin's father remained firm in his beliefs, he was receptive to not sharing these statements in front of Justin.

Case Study #2

16-year-old "Alyssa" sought therapy for stress and anxiety. Alyssa possessed extreme fear surrounding food, weight and body image. Alyssa's parents were concerned, and frequently told Alyssa she had a beautiful body and did not need to worry. Alyssa's parents did not force diets or exercise upon Alyssa. Instead, they were supportive and loving.

After a few therapy sessions, Alyssa disclosed that her mother was highly critical of her own body. Alyssa's mother frequently looked in the mirror stating, "Ugh, I'm too fat, I hate how much weight I've gained, I need to work out more." Alyssa's mother had no idea her own self-judgments and criticisms were projected onto Alyssa. From hearing her mother's words, Alyssa feared that she would become unworthy if she were to gain weight.

Through individual and family therapy, Alyssa was able to communicate her feelings to her mother. Alyssa did not blame her mother, but instead shared how confusing and upsetting it was to hear her mother's self-judgments. Alyssa's mother was receptive to Alyssa's comments and stopped disparaging herself in front of Alyssa. Alyssa's mother also used this feedback as an opportunity to start her own individual therapy. In examining her own self-judgment, Alyssa's mother helped Alyssa, as well as herself. **These examples demonstrate how judgments are often unintentionally harmful to teenagers. Consider your own judgments and the ways in which judgments can be modified into constructive conversations.**

CHAPTER 7

Self-Worth: Boundaries Over Restrictions

As a therapist, I believe self-worth to be the ultimate weapon in combating anxiety. A strong sense of self-worth is like going into battle with a suit of indestructible armor. No matter what is thrown at an individual, the armor deflects any form of attack. Attacks simply bounce off the armor and protect them from injury or harm. Similarly, self-worth is armor in fighting any form of attack from anxiety. A strong sense of self-worth guides an individual to persevere and move forward.

Self-Worth: The Ultimate Weapon

I personally define self-worth as the belief in one's own ability and strength. When an individual has strong self-worth, they navigate life more freely and with ease. This is not to state an individual with strong self-worth never feels sad, angry or hurt. Instead, strong self-worth helps depersonalize negative feelings and practice self-compassion. Negativity or unkindness toward oneself has little positive effect, particularly among teenagers.

People often correlate low self-worth in teenagers with depression. In simplified terms, when teenagers feel bad about themselves, they become sad and depressed. While this can be true, low self-worth can also create or increase anxiety. Generally speaking, anxiety is a fear-based feeling; fear of a catastrophic event, fear of failure, fear of judgment, fear of ridicule, fear of unsafe situations, fear of the unknown. The list of fears goes on and on and can become highly imaginative. With this in mind, many anxiety-based beliefs center upon the fear of "not being good enough."

When teenagers strengthen their self-worth, they begin to regard themselves as "good enough." Feeling good enough significantly supports teenagers in peacefully navigating adolescence. When teens begin to trust and believe in themselves, they can confidently face their fears. Enhanced self-worth lifts teenagers back up after challenges, thus reducing the fear of failure. Overall, strong self-worth serves as a guide through social and emotional stress. Most importantly, self-worth becomes a crucial tool that teens can use for the rest of their lives, throughout college, the workforce and into adulthood.

Sadly, very few teenagers are aware of concepts such as self-worth, self-compassion or self-love. Most are highly critical of themselves, which is why criticism from their parents hurt even more. For the majority of adolescents, any form of hardship becomes a direct reflection of their self-worth. Reference the two examples below:

Example #1

A teenager is rejected by a peer or romantic interest. Typically, the teenager internalizes the rejection.

The teenager most likely thinks, "It is because I'm not pretty enough." (Or handsome, sexy, funny, or smart enough.) The teenager rarely thinks, "That rejection hurts my feelings, but that is not the right partner or friend for me."

Example #2

Despite studying, a teenager fails a test. Often, this becomes a reflection of their self-worth.

The teenager most likely responds, "I am a bad student. I am so stupid." The teenager is unlikely to respond, "Wow, that was really hard, and I felt bad receiving an F. However, the material was really challenging, and I am going to talk to my teacher to see what I can do to improve."

These examples illustrate the effects of strong self-worth on teenage anxiety. When a teenager's self-worth is low, they are more likely to become anxious after facing adversity. However, when a teenager's self-worth is high, they can depersonalize the hardship and easily bounce back.

Self-Love and Self-Acceptance

The power of self-worth might be easy for an adult to comprehend. However, building self-worth in teenagers can be challenging, and does not occur overnight. For most teens, the concept of self-worth or self-love feels foreign and unachievable. If your teenager's self-esteem is particularly low, it is helpful to begin with self-acceptance. Self-acceptance centers upon approving of one's self in a more neutral stance.

The next section provides four concrete steps to enhance your teenager's self-acceptance and self-worth.

Boundaries Over Restrictions

Step 1: Speak with Your Teenager Like a Teenager

> "I just want my parents to stop treating me like I'm eight years old. I know I'm not an adult but I'm not a kid anymore."
>
> **−14-YEAR-OLD CLIENT**

Speaking with your teenager like a teenager can sound like an odd idea. You might still regard your teen as a child, particularly if they are a younger teen (age 13 or 14). Your teenager might still retain some child-like features or possess similar interests to when they were younger. If this is the case, it is still important to remember your teenager is no longer a child. Your acceptance of this change heightens your teenager's self-worth and self-acceptance.

It can be difficult for parents to accept that their child is now a teenager, and it is common to feel a loss in this realization. Moreover, it is healthy to grieve your teenager's child-like state. Processing your grief in a constructive manner leads to the acceptance of your teenager becoming an adolescent. Progressing from childhood to adolescence is a natural part of the life cycle. However, preventing your teen from emotionally transitioning to adolescence is destructive for their self-worth. We will explore this concept more in Step 2.

When you are ready to start accepting your teenager's adolescence, begin speaking with your teenager like a teenager. This can be confusing for many parents who are unsure how to communicate with a teenager. As a reminder, no longer speak with your teenager like a child you have to control and constantly monitor. While your teenager is not yet a full-grown adult, your teenager is beginning to possess adult emotions.

Consider the emotional qualities we value as adults that can be applied to teenagers. Listening, validation and non-judgmental feedback are generally more appreciated than micromanagement, control or judgment. Begin incorporating communication tools such as listening and appropriate validation in order to enhance your teenager's self-worth. Show your teenager you no longer view them as a child, but more as an evolving young adult. By lessening control, you demonstrate respect for your teenager. Your teenager will begin to feel confident in their decisions and will respect you for respecting them. Moreover, your teenager will start to value your insight and feel safe in your support.

Step 2: Restrict Your Restrictions

"I feel like my parents' strict nature just completely backfired. They didn't let me do anything when I was in high school, and I completely went off the deep end as soon as I got into college. I found myself using drugs, having unprotected sex, and just going wild."

–22-YEAR-OLD CLIENT

Prior to moving onto Step 2, it is crucial that you feel comfortable with Step 1. Step 2 can feel scary for many caring parents. In fact, it is common for parents to seek their own counseling while embracing this next step.

Unhealthy restrictions control your teenager's life. Restrictions entail telling your teenager what to do and what not to do. Restrictions prohibit natural activities, actions, and events from occurring in your teenager's life. Unhealthy restrictions are authoritative, punitive and can cause your teenager to sneak, lie and deceive.

Furthermore, restrictions dominate your teenager and are highly detrimental to their self-esteem. Unfortunately, unhealthy restrictions can be subjective and difficult to identify.

Here are a few common ways parents negatively restrict their teens:

- Not allowing socialization with friends
- Prohibiting dating
- Controlling who your teenager dates
- Telling your teenager they cannot attend parties
- Threatening punishment if your teenager is to drink, smoke or have sex
- Constantly rescuing your teenager from making mistakes or enabling

If you are guilty of the above behavior, you are not alone. Highly protective, concerned and loving parents can be the most restrictive. Restrictive parents often have positive intentions and believe they are saving their teenager from hardship. However, restrictions result in the opposite of heightened self-worth. Restrictions lower self-esteem and teach your teenager they cannot make decisions for themself. Restrictions convey a lack of trust in your teenager, as well as a lack of respect. Additionally, restrictions keep your teenager in a child-like state.

There are emergency situations where restrictions are necessary. These are extreme scenarios in which your teenager's safety is truly at risk. If you are uncertain, be on the side of caution and consult with a mental health professional. When there is a clear safety concern, it is understandable to impose restrictions. For example, it is appropriate to restrict your teenager from dating an individual who is a threat to their safety (e.g., someone significantly older, involved in criminal activity, etc.).

Step 3: Set Boundaries

In restricting your restrictions, I am not advising you to allow your teenager to run wild. A teenager who is completely unsupervised can be just as anxious as a restricted teenager. Teenagers benefit from structure, and an emotional safety net helps provide a sense of security. Teenagers need to feel supported while learning how to make decisions, but still in control of their own lives. Instead of unfairly restricting your teen, learn to set healthy, realistic boundaries.

You might now be asking, what are the differences between boundaries and restrictions, and how can I differentiate the two? Boundaries are safe, healthy, realistic and appropriate limits. Boundaries provide security while still allowing your teenager to learn from their experiences. Restrictions are prohibitive, confining, and do not leave room for growth. To better understand the difference between restrictions and boundaries, consider the following examples:

Example #1

Your 16-year-old son would like to attend a party thrown by a peer. You fear there will be alcohol at the party.

Boundary: You let your son attend the party. However, you inform your son that he cannot drive if he consumes any alcohol.

Potential consequences of boundary:

- Your son attends the party and does not drink.
- Your son attends the party and drinks but returns home via Uber or Lyft.
- Your son attends the party, drinks and drives. You then determine an appropriate disciplinary action (grounding, extra chores). Your son learns from his mistake in an appropriate manner.

Both scenarios A and B result in your teen's respect for you, as well as appreciation and trust in their own decision-making abilities. Scenario C provides an appropriate consequence to the boundary violation.
Restriction: You prohibit your son from attending the party.

Potential consequences of restriction:

- Your son sneaks out of the house or lies in order to attend the party.

- Your son drinks and drives.

- Your son stays home, resents your control and feels you treat him like a child.

Please note how all of these scenarios are *negative*.

Example #2

Your 17-year-old daughter wants to date a classmate. You worry your teenager will be sexually active within this new relationship.

Boundary: You allow your daughter to date the classmate but speak about the importance of contraception.

Potential consequences of boundary:

- Your daughter practices safe sex.

- Your daughter does not practice safe sex and deals with the repercussions.

Scenario A results in your teen's respect for you in trusting her decision-making abilities. Scenario B is unlikely unless your daughter does not adhere to contraceptive methods.

Restriction: You prohibit your daughter from dating.

Potential consequences of restriction:

- Your daughter dates and has sex without you knowing.
- Your daughter does not practice safe sex and does not use contraception.

Note how all of the scenarios above are negative. While these examples may sound extreme, these situations are not uncommon. Healthy boundaries prompt learning from mistakes, while restrictions lead to lying and deceit. Boundaries elicit safety and security while building self-esteem, while restrictions stunt healthy and natural adolescent development.

Step 4: Do *Not* Rescue

> "I'm terrified to move away from home and start college. I hate to say it, but my parents bail me out of everything. They have even done homework for me, emailed teachers asking for extensions, and pushed for me to not take tests. I don't think

that will work in college. The thought of having to actually do things on my own is terrifying."

–17-YEAR-OLD CLIENT

In setting boundaries, it is crucial not to rescue your teenager from their mistakes. It is healthy for your teen to learn from their mistakes, provided they are not jeopardizing their safety. Rescuing your teenager leads to enabling behaviors and ultimately negatively impacts their self-esteem. Learning from mistakes is excellent for self-esteem: it builds resilience and strength, rather than dependence and victimization.

Instead of rescuing, frame mistakes as lessons and opportunities for growth. Learning, rather than rescuing, teaches your teenager that it is okay to be an imperfect person. Allow your teen to metaphorically scrape their knees and heal. This is an opportunity for you to have a teaching moment as a parent; teach your teenager they can "fail" and still be lovable. To clarify, examples of rescuing behaviors versus opportunities for learning are listed below:

Example #1

Your 15-year-old would like to attend a concert on a school night. You allow them to attend, but your teenager stays out late and would like to skip school the next day.

Rescuing: You call the school and forge a doctor's note stating your teenager is sick.

Consequence: Your teenager learns that you will bail them out and they can ignore responsibilities.

Learning: You insist your teenager attend school the next day despite their tired state.

Consequence: Your teenager learns to stay home on a school night due to responsibilities.

Example #2

Your 13-year-old would like to attend a weekend trip away with their friend and their friend's family. Your teen has a test first period Monday morning. You allow them to attend the trip and advise them to study either before or during the time away. Your teenager attends the trip but ignores your advice to study and fails the test.

Rescuing: You email your teenager's teacher asking for a retake of the test.

Consequence: Your teenager learns you will enable irresponsible behavior, and they can overlook their academic responsibilities.

Learning: You suggest your teenager speak with their teacher about extra credit opportunities and encourage learning from the experience.

Consequence: Your teenager learns time management and to prioritize responsibilities.

Of course, there are specific situations in which it is appropriate to help your teenager. If your child is in danger, it is wise to rescue, rather than frame the opportunity for learning. However, be mindful of constant rescuing and enabling behavior. Rescuing and enabling might appear insignificant in the moment, but can cause serious long-term effects. Remember, learning and resilience are crucial in building self-esteem and lessening anxiety. Refraining from rescuing is not easy and can go against your instincts as a parent. Be patient with yourself during the process and seek your own support if necessary.

CHAPTER 8

Leading by Example

> "My parents have always gone to therapy and also go to 12-step meetings. I never had an issue about going to therapy myself or getting my own support because my parents do the same."
>
> —17-YEAR-OLD CLIENT

Leading by example is a subtle, yet powerful technique you can utilize as a parent. Leading by example requires no engagement or partnership from your teenager, and you can start the process immediately. Most importantly, leading by example will benefit the emotional wellness of your teenager, as well as yourself.

Overt Support vs Covert Support

Leading by example can be forgotten by even the most thoughtful parents. After all, your role as a parent often involves placing your child's needs before your own. This is a kind, selfless, and loving gesture that might be instinctual for you. In order to fully grasp this notion, reflect back to when your teenager was a baby. If your teenager was adopted after infancy, envision the first few months after the adoption.

Consider the ways in which you placed your baby's needs before your own. This was a time when you demonstrated "overt" support. You might have sacrificed sleep to ensure your baby was fed and cared for. You might not have prioritized self-care, as your baby was entirely dependent on you for survival. If you had not placed your baby's needs first, and demonstrated overt support, the outcomes could have been disastrous. Your baby could have suffered, and your role was to prioritize your baby's needs.

Now, consider the present time and envision your baby as the teenager they are today.

Ask yourself the following questions:

- Do I still embody the same mentality as when my child was a baby?

- Am I showing myself self-care now that my child is not entirely dependent on me?

- Am I teaching my teenager the importance of attending to my own emotional needs?

- What messages am I sending about self-care?

- How am I leading my child by example in regard to mental health?

- How can I show my teenager that I care for them by also taking care of myself?

Please note, I am not encouraging you to disregard your teenager's needs and well-being. Rather, I am prompting you to modify the ways in which you place your teenager's needs first. Instead, lead by example and allow your teenager to witness you caring for your own emotional well-being. You can view leading by example as a way of demonstrating "covert," or more subtle support. There are many ways to demonstrate covert support for your teenager. To begin, we will address caring for your own mental health.

Covert Support #1: Your Own Emotional Support

A simple way to demonstrate covert support is to lead by example through seeking your own emotional support. Your emotional support could be in the form of individual therapy, counseling, workshops, seminars and so forth. This highly effective action subtly teaches your teenager to follow in your footsteps, and develop an acceptance surrounding mental health support.

Unfortunately, I often receive resistance when I highlight the importance of emotional support for parents.

I am met with phrases such as:

- "I understand the idea but I just don't have time for my own therapy."
- "My schedule is too busy to go to a workshop or seminar."
- "I can't afford counseling right now."
- "I am too preoccupied helping my kid to find myself a therapist."
- "I don't need help, it's my teenager that has the issue."

These are common reactions from parents who are accustomed to placing their child's needs first. These parents have no issue putting their own mental health needs to the side, and are more comfortable providing overt support to their teenager. However, when parents help themselves emotionally, they also help their teenagers.

We can illustrate this concept with the frequently referenced oxygen mask analogy. On a flight prior to take off, the flight attendants will state, "In case of emergency, put on your own oxygen mask before helping others." This is accompanied by a video of a parent placing their own oxygen mask on themself, before assisting their child.

The oxygen mask analogy is excellent in regard to parenting and teenage mental health. When you are neglecting your own emotional needs, it can be difficult to help your teenager. When you are stressed, depressed or anxious yourself, how can you support someone else who is anxious? On the contrary, when you care for your own emotional wellbeing, you lead by example. In leading by example, you can be fully present and resourceful for your teenager.

Interestingly, this concept was emphasized on my first day of graduate school for social work. The most helpful advice I received during my therapist training was to practice self-care by attending therapy. While most of the parents reading this book have little intention of becoming a therapist, being a parent of an anxious teenager can be a full-time and exhausting job. I highly recommend beginning your own therapy to help both yourself and your teenager.

Case Study

16-year-old "Alex" came to therapy for anxiety. During our first session, Alex expressed shame in seeking therapeutic support. Alex thought therapy was for the "weak and broken." Fortunately, Alex maintained an open mind and was willing to give therapy a chance. After several months, Alex informed me that his parents were opposed to visiting a therapist themselves.

Alex felt confused as to why he should engage in therapy, when his parents were resistant to their own therapy. When Alex shared these feelings with his parents, he was met with phrases such as, "I can deal with things on my own," or "we don't need therapy, we don't have anxiety like you." While unintentional, this sent mixed messages surrounding the value of therapy.

While Alex's parents remained resistant to their own support, Alex fortunately began to notice a decrease in his anxiety. However, Alex frequently expressed the desire for his parents to have their own level of support, and change their narrative surrounding therapy.

Covert Support #2: Other Forms of Self-Care

> "I learned my self-care practices from my mom. She always made art to help her relax. When I was younger, I used to copy her, and I ended up getting into the routine of making art to relax too. It just stuck with me and I really like it."
>
> —13-YEAR-OLD CLIENT

Have you given much thought to your own self-care practices? Many of my clients' parents roll their eyes when I ask this question. The term "self-care" is often referenced very casually, and its value can be lost. Just as people are resistant to attending individual therapy, you might feel there is not enough time, money or purpose in regular self-care. However, your personal self-care teaches your teenager to practice their own self-care.

Self-care can manifest differently for each person. Your self-care could be daily meditation, exercise and walks in nature. For another individual, self-care might be cooking a delicious meal, making art or journaling. Acts of self-care can also change with age and time. As a teenager, my self-care was going to punk rock concerts where the singer was screaming into a microphone. Now, as an adult, my self-care is practicing yoga, engaging in a creative hobby and reading a novel with a hot cup of tea. It is perfectly acceptable for self-care routines to change and evolve over the lifespan, but self-care ideally restores your emotional wellness.

Unfortunately, most people do not practice regular self-care, and when they do, they feel guilt or shame. Have you ever thought, "I should be doing something else," instead of practicing self-care? Perhaps you have even said this statement out loud or prevented yourself from engaging in a constructive act of self-care. While it is necessary to still attend to responsibilities, learn to prioritize regular acts of self-care. Moreover, be mindful of any feelings of guilt or shame you experience when engaging in an act of self-care.

There are numerous benefits from practicing regular self-care. In my private practice, the clients who engage in regular self-care have less stress and anxiety than the clients who do not practice regular self-care. Interestingly, I have noticed this pattern among both my teenage and adult clients. A routine of consistent self-care throughout adolescence leads to healthy habits in adulthood. Self-care is a useful tool teenagers can utilize in the present, as well as in the future.

When you *do not* practice your own self-care, you can unintentionally teach your teenager to neglect their own self-care. However, when your teenager witnesses you caring for yourself, your teenager understands they can do the same. Your teenager learns it is not only acceptable but also encouraged to care for their mental health.

Covert Support #3: Your Own Self-Esteem and Boundaries

In the previous chapter we discussed the importance of your teenager's self-esteem. Hopefully, you are supportive of your teenager's process in building self-esteem and are now setting non-restrictive boundaries. In leading by example, reflect on your own, personal self-esteem. Do you treat yourself with love through setting boundaries with others, accepting and approving of yourself, and practicing self-care? Or do you question, doubt or put yourself down? Overall, are you leading by example in building high self-esteem?

If your answers lean toward the negative, do not judge, but commend yourself for becoming aware. Western culture typically does not encourage high self-esteem and healthy boundaries. Instead, we are taught to tell ourselves we are not good enough. Additionally, there are few traditional educational classes that teach us to develop healthy self-esteem or strong boundary setting skills. Perhaps you were also raised in a family, community or culture where the people surrounding you had low self-esteem and poor boundaries. It might have felt normal for you to grow up not liking yourself.

With this in mind, make an effort to improve your own self-esteem. Engage in this process for your own mental health, as well as for the mental health of your teenager. If you have never prioritized your own self-esteem and set boundaries, now is the time. It is never too late to start caring for yourself, and sometimes you need a little motivation. If your teenager is struggling, allow their struggles to be a motivator for your self-improvement. You can help your teenager through leading by example by increasing your self-esteem and setting boundaries.

Self-esteem and boundaries are complex issues, and therefore do not expect rapid, overnight changes. If your self-esteem is particularly low or in need of significant improvement, seek professional guidance from a therapist or counselor. Additionally, attend support groups, seminars and engage in other forms of holistic healing. For more information, reference the list of alternative forms of support provided in Chapter 11.

The Observant Teen

Teenagers are observant and impressionable creatures. Leading by example is an act your teenager will notice, either on a conscious or subconscious level. While your teenager might not express outward appreciation, leading by example sends a powerful message. Openness to your own emotional support could affect whether your teenager is willing to receive support themself. Your personal self-care teaches your teenager to prioritize their personal wellness. Lastly, your own self-esteem and ability to set boundaries paves the path for your teenager's mental health. Remember, you are modeling behavior for your teenager.

PART III

Additional Support

CHAPTER 9

Seeking Support

"Therapy has really helped me overcome my anxiety. Even though I still get worried and scared sometimes, I know I can handle stress and that everything will be okay."

—14-YEAR-OLD CLIENT

Sometimes the information discussed in the previous chapters is simply not enough to help your teenager. This is understandable given the complex nature of anxiety. Even with the information provided, I still recommend speaking with your teenager about seeking therapy or counseling. In doing so, it is of utmost importance to refrain from forcing your teenager to attend therapy as punishment. Additionally, do not insist that your teenager work with a therapist they do not like.

Encouraging, Not Forcing

Forcing treatment from a particular therapist can be disastrous and leaves the concept of therapy like a bitter taste in their mouth. It is essential to avoid this so your teenager can remain open to therapy later in life.

In my current practice, I treat many adult clients who were once opposed to meeting with a therapist. I see this often in couples, when a partner resists marital or couples counseling because they were "forced to go to therapy" by their parents when they were a teenager. Many adults struggle due to resistance stemming from experiences in therapy during childhood. Therefore, allow therapy to be a place of refuge for your teenager, not a setting for punishment and additional stress.

Searching and Shopping

Finding an appropriate therapist often entails your teenager not seeing the same therapist as you or another family member. If you and your teen have already attended family therapy together, it might be more comfortable for your teenager to work with a separate therapist. Many teenagers feel fine working with the same therapist as you, their siblings, or even their family therapist. However, a separate therapist can offer a fresh, unbiased perspective. Have a conversation with your teenager as to what feels most appropriate.

This process might also include "shopping" for a therapist. Allow your teenager to visit different therapists until they decide it is an appropriate fit. This process can be similar to searching for a doctor who makes you feel comfortable. It can take time and might require several visits to different practitioners before finding a match. Since therapy is tremendously personal and can be uncomfortable at times, it is imperative for your teenager to like their therapist.

Place yourself in your teenager's frame of mind when searching for a therapist. Ask yourself, how would you want to find a therapist if you were seeking your own personal therapy? Most likely, you would not want a therapist chosen for you by someone else. You might want to meet with a variety of different professionals before selecting one that resonates with you.

Remember, establishing rapport with a therapist can be a process, and your teen might not feel comfortable right away. It is natural for your teenager to feel nervous about therapy, and it can even require a few sessions before they begin to feel comfortable. However, if your teenager expresses complete terror, fear, or dread about going back to a therapist, I implore you to listen. It is crucial your teenager feels heard and respected. Do not push your teenager to work with a specific therapist when they feel it is not a good match.

An Open Therapy Dialogue

Once you and your teenager have begun actively searching for a therapist, engage in another detailed and open conversation. In this conversation, ask your teenager what they are looking for in a therapist. You and your teenager can examine what they hope to "find" in a therapist and explore logistics in order to specify your search. There are many therapists, and it can be overwhelming to search without narrowing down criteria.

I suggest asking your teenager some of the following questions:

- Would you prefer to see a therapist with the same gender as you?

- How about the same ethnicity or racial background?

- Would you prefer to work with someone younger or someone older?

- Would you feel comfortable seeing someone in person or virtually?

- Would you be open to "traditional" talk therapy or would you prefer to find someone who specializes in some form of art/movement or creative therapy?

- Is there a specific specialization you would be interested in? (e.g., working with someone who specializes in the LGBTQ+ population, adoption, etc.)

- What would feel best for you and how can I help you feel comfortable while we search?

In my own therapy practice, I am very selective about the clients I work with. This is to ensure an appropriate fit and to facilitate eventual openness. A qualified therapist will be direct with you right from the start. If the therapist feels your teenager is not the best fit, they will most likely refer them to someone else.

Many therapists have different areas of expertise and specializations. If your teenager has concerns in addition to anxiety, find a therapist knowledgeable in that field. For example, if your teenager struggles with alcohol use as well as anxiety, research therapists who specialize in treating both anxiety and substance use disorders.

Specifications

"I really enjoy variation in my therapy sessions. I like that sometimes we go for walks, sometimes we do art, and sometimes we sit in the office and just talk."

—16-YEAR-OLD CLIENT

Some teenagers flourish working with a therapist who provides alternative treatments in conjunction with traditional talk therapy. Art therapy, music therapy, and even movement or walking therapy can be interesting avenues to explore. With consent from you as a parent, some therapists offer services outside of the office, such as an outdoor area in their building or at a park. This might appear a bit unconventional, but it can be helpful to consider. These are also valuable options if your teenager is resistant to traditional psychotherapy.

If your teenager continues to express resistance, and you have financial flexibility, you might consider a "home visit" therapist. Many private practice therapists offer this service for an additional cost. Home visit therapy sessions can be a safe way for a client to ease into therapy. Home visits allow therapy to be held in a comfortable setting, where the teenager feels more relaxed and at ease. If your teenager has experienced serious trauma, this can be a wise choice due to familiarity with the home setting. Many of my home visit clients report feeling supported by the presence of their pets during our sessions, as well as knowing their parents are in the next room.

If you and your teenager decide a home visit therapist is best, it is of utmost importance for your teen to have privacy during sessions. Needless to say, avoid interruptions and limit distractions by turning off electronics and reducing noise in the neighboring rooms. Comfort and privacy are absolutely essential for successful home visit sessions.

Whichever avenue of therapy your teenager decides to pursue, engage in extensive research. Find a therapist who is knowledgeable in adolescent mental health and has experience treating teenagers with anxiety. Your teenager's school counselor or doctor will most likely have a list of therapy referrals for you, or you can reference www.psychologytoday.com, which provides a directory of therapists in your area.

Payment and Cost

Remain open to therapy even if you have financial constraints or limited funds. If you have insurance, you can research therapists within your provider network, where paying cash out of pocket is not required. Additionally, many mental health centers often employ trainees or associates who are not yet fully licensed but offer low or sliding scale fees. These trainees are required to complete a number of clinical hours under the supervision of a qualified professional. Although still in training, associates can possess the dedication, energy, and passion to provide excellent services. Welcome the idea of your teenager working with a trainee or associate. In fact, I treated many teenagers while I was an associate under supervision.

Another option for low-cost therapy services is a charity or non-profit group. Several non-profit organizations offer low-cost or free therapy services from highly qualified individuals. Many therapists in private practice engage in pro bono work for these organizations as a way of giving back. Additionally, many "cash pay" therapists offer sliding scale payment options for clients. It is appropriate to ask a therapist if they work with clients on a sliding scale basis. The practitioner can then determine if and how the request can be accommodated.

Alternate Options

If your teenager continues to express complete opposition to therapy or does not like any of the therapists they see, seek another form of support. I regularly collaborate with life coaches in my practice and find that coaching can often feel less threatening and scary for teens. Several of my own clients sought therapy only after, or in conjunction with, working alongside a life coach. Many of these clients recall feeling more "warmed up" to therapy after working with a life coach.

I will be very clear that life coaching is not the same as therapy. Coaching often addresses the "here and now" rather than delving deep into childhood experiences or family dynamics. Many coaches operate in a more casual and relaxed manner with their clients, which can ease teenagers into the idea of receiving support. Some coaches do not conduct sessions in a clinical office, but rather over the phone or at a coffee shop, park, or other casual setting. Overall, this is more common in coaching practices rather than traditional therapy.

Coaching can be an excellent form of support for teens due to its natural and organic nature. Coaching might remind your teenager of spending time with a mentor who has a plethora of guidance and knowledge. If your teenager agrees to pursue coaching, they have taken an amazing step in their healing. You can still consider therapy as an option for the future or whenever your teenager is ready. However, do not discredit the healing powers of effective life coaching. Much like searching for a therapist, it is crucial to search for a coach who is certified in their field and is a good fit for your teenager.

When appropriate, it can also be helpful to seek specific support groups for your teenager. Many non-profit groups offer community events or supportive environments through online forums. If your teenager struggles with any substance use issues in conjunction with anxiety, I suggest twelve-step recovery groups. There are many twelve-step groups that specifically welcome teenagers and young adults, such as Young

Peoples' Alcoholics Anonymous. If you or anyone else close to your teenager has struggled with substances, Ala-Teen can also be a helpful resource. Ala-Teen mirrors the framework of Al-Anon, a support group for loved ones of those with addiction, but focuses on adolescent participation.

There are numerous other types of support groups, such as grief processing and eating disorder recovery. Many of these groups also offer online meetings, which can provide additional comfort and anonymity. Overall, support groups are a wonderful way for your teenager to establish connection and guidance. Additionally, most meetings and support groups are completely free of charge.

Another form of additional support might be religious or spiritual counseling for your teenager. Only pursue this path if your teenager already identifies with a faith or spiritual path, and it is not forced. Refrain from pushing your own religious beliefs onto your teenager if it does not resonate. While you can share your beliefs, be respectful of your teen's perceptions of religion and spirituality.

If your teenager is open to spiritual or religious counseling, but opposed to therapy, consider this option. Spiritual counseling can be a fantastic way for your teenager to feel comfort and safety in having faith in a higher being. I have witnessed enormous success in my clients who use their faith as a coping mechanism. Moreover, many religious and spiritual counseling centers offer free or low-cost services.

Above all, speak with your teenager about what feels right to them. The alternative options listed above are not the same as individual psychotherapy, but still provide helpful mentorship and guidance. These resources can guide your teenager to feel safe in communicating their feelings. These forms of support also offer a space of healing outside of the family and immediate peer group. Furthermore, any type of healthy support can lead teenagers to be more open to therapy later in life.

Case Study

After a few short-term school counseling sessions, it became clear that Brenden was struggling with anxiety and depression. For various reasons, Brenden's parents were opposed to seeking therapy with a private clinician outside of school. Brenden's family culture tended to stigmatize therapy, and therefore, long- term counseling was not an option.

Fortunately, Brenden and his parents were open to other forms of support. Brenden and his family were religious, and believed in spiritual counseling. While faith-based counseling and individual therapy differ in many ways, Brenden was able to find relief in speaking with a spiritual leader. Brenden became more involved in his church, attended youth groups, and found new mentors to confide in. Brenden's mental health improved with this support outside of school.

Psychiatry

A pivotal component of additional support might involve psychiatry or medication. This is often a tricky topic for many parents. There can be a stigma with medication, and it is natural for parents to be hesitant to place a developing teenager on medication. Psychiatric medications have also significantly changed throughout the years, and parents might be unsure about the side effects. However, medication can be a crucial and even life-changing form of mental health support.

First and foremost, remember the biological factors contributing to teenage anxiety. Often, there truly are chemical imbalances and genetic influences that can be treated with medication. Instead of ruling out a medical intervention, maintain an open mindset surrounding medication. Your teenager could be just as confused about psychiatry and will look to you for support.

The process of searching for a psychiatrist often begins with your teenager's therapist contacting you, their client's parent. Unless your teenager's therapist is a medical doctor, they are not qualified to state if medication is required and cannot prescribe medications. However, your teenager's therapist can provide referrals for psychiatrists if they feel your teenager would benefit from an evaluation. If your teenager's therapist recommends a psychiatric evaluation, listen. This is of utmost importance, as most therapists will not recommend psychiatric evaluations for minors unless deemed necessary.

Ignoring a psychiatry referral can be extremely detrimental. Due to fear or confusion, parents might be inclined to ignore referrals, which can only cause more hardship for your teen. If you have questions as to why a psychiatric evaluation would be helpful, contact your teenager's therapist. If the therapist has not reached out to you about psychiatric referrals, it is most likely that they feel an evaluation is not necessary. However, if you are concerned, have a discussion with your teenager's therapist. If your teenager is regular with therapy, and shows signs of improvement, psychiatry might not be necessary.

As a whole, remain open to various options while seeking additional support for your teenager. Support might appear differently for your teenager than for you, and it is important to respect their process. We will explore how to continue to show support in the following chapters.

CHAPTER 10

Receiving Help

> "I know things are better now that my teen is getting some help, but it's really hard for me to take my hands off the steering wheel. What else can I do?"
>
> —Parent of a 14-year-old client

Perhaps with a little encouragement, your teenager is open to additional support and begins attending therapy on a regular basis. You might feel as though you can finally breathe again, and as if a hundred pounds has been lifted from your shoulders. Your teenager might even start to show initial signs of improvement. However, what comes next? How do you continue to help your teenager? The steps listed in the next two chapters are guidelines for when your teenager begins to receive help.

Step 1: Respect and Encourage

The first and most important step is to express respect and credit your teenager for their decision to attend therapy. Mental health issues can be overwhelming for teens, and their courage deserves to be acknowledged. Teenagers, as well as adults, can struggle with this initial step in caring for their mental health.

Your teenager might not admit this directly, but your encouragement and validation can provide a sense of safety and relief. While the widespread perception of therapy and mental health might be positively shifting, many teenagers begin therapy feeling "broken" or "problematic." This is another reason why I discourage sending your teenager to therapy as a form of punishment. It is critical that your teenager feels your support in perceiving therapy as an act of positivity and strength, rather than a sign of weakness.

While this is important for all teenagers, I have noticed the significance of emphasizing this sentiment to male adolescents. Sadly, many teenage males still embody cultural beliefs of being "emotionally strong" and "to figure things out on their own." Vulnerability can often be confused with weakness, and therapy can be highly emotionally vulnerable. If your teenager begins therapy without the benefit of your encouragement or respect, they can continue to believe they are weak, broken, or not good enough. However, when you acknowledge their strength, they can begin to view themselves in a new and improved light.

When applicable and if possible, it is helpful for both parents to verbalize respect, support, and encouragement. Very often, a teenager will possess one supportive parent, while the other parent perceives therapy as unnecessary and an additional expense. Envision the amount of confusion and increased anxiety this can cause for your teenager. Several teenage clients in my practice began therapy with mixed feelings due to varying parental perspectives.

Conflicted emotions can arise about which parent has the correct view surrounding therapy. Not only does this cause more stress for a teenager, but it can also elicit feelings of resentment and anger toward their parents. If you and your teenager's other parent hold diametrically opposed points of view about your teenager's therapy, consider seeking your own counseling. Parental approval, encouragement, and support are crucial in helping your teenager.

Overall, express pride in your teenager's choice to take care of themself emotionally. Reinforce beliefs that vulnerability is a sign of strength, and emphasize the positive and healing nature of therapy.

Step 2: Foster Independence

"Therapy is the one place I can speak honestly and freely."

—13-YEAR-OLD CLIENT

Perhaps it was not terribly difficult for you to encourage and respect your teenager for attending therapy. You might love the idea of your teenager working with a therapist and want to help more. The second step of supporting your teenager, is fostering independence by avoiding force and intrusion, can be difficult for many parents.

Teenage Therapy Exercise: Visualization

To begin this step, complete the Teenage Therapy Visualization Exercise below. Once again, envision yourself as an adolescent. You can review your answers from Chapter 4 as a reminder.

How did you look physically? How did you feel emotionally? What was your support system like? Consider the ups and downs you experienced as a teenager.

As you imagine yourself as a teenager, envision yourself talking to a therapist about your deepest and darkest secrets. Some of the secrets might be shameful or emotionally painful to share. Imagine yourself feeling relieved and safe, as you converse with someone who has no connection to anyone else in your life. Feel the trust you have with this person, knowing the thoughts you share will remain private and undisclosed to others.

Now, imagine that your parents would like to come into this safe space you have cultivated. Envision discovering that your parents called your therapist numerous times, perhaps without you knowing. You then learn that your parents asked for advice on how to "deal" with you and asked questions that make you feel like you need to be "fixed." You also find out that your parents spoke about their own issues with your therapist and would like to use them as their own personal therapist. Let yourself sit with this and feel what comes up for you.

Finally, imagine your parents now insisting on entering your safe space regularly. Your parents demand to know what you have learned from the conversations with your therapist and what tools you have acquired. Hear your parents say they would like to bring other members of your family into the sessions, perhaps even your siblings. Picture your parents wanting to know details about your conversations in therapy. Imagine your parents coming to therapy with you, even though you do not want them in attendance.

What emotions arise when envisioning this situation? Consider how you would feel about your parents, siblings, and even yourself. What would make you more comfortable? Keep your answers in mind as you read the following section.

The Importance of Privacy, Alone Time and Independence

The situation described above has occurred numerous times in my therapy practice. I frequently receive nervous calls from parents of my teenage clients. This is understandable, as parents are concerned and would like answers. They want updates, solutions for problematic behaviors, and strategies to help address larger issues through family therapy. These parents might also be spending a significant amount of money on their teenager's therapy and would like to know how their teenager benefits from services. Parents would like to ensure their teenager is well taken care of. Therefore, you might be asking; why wouldn't an involved parent phone their teenager's therapist weekly or insist on family therapy with the same therapist?

The answer is simple: *to respect your teenager's privacy and foster independence.*

Reference the visualization exercise you just completed. Didn't it feel positive to have privacy and a safe space? Chances are, your teenager feels the same and enjoys alone time in therapy. Although teenagers are minors, they want to feel independent. Again, reflect back to when you were a teen. Did you enjoy your independence? How about now as an adult? Did you, and do you still, like time to yourself, even if you adore your family and the people around you? Sometimes we need time and space apart from the people we love to feel authentic and replenished. Furthermore, independence can increase self-esteem and improve the quality of our relationships. This is especially relevant for teenagers, who are in the process of forming and understanding their own sense of self.

The Ability to be Independent

> "I'm terrified I won't be able to do things without my parents helping me. They do everything for me."
>
> —15-YEAR-OLD CLIENT

Respecting your teenager's therapy shows you trust and have faith in their ability to be independent. Teens are forming their sense of self, and often test their abilities to function as newly independent individuals. Many of my teenage clients identify the source of their anxiety as the failure of independence. This can manifest in anxieties related to school, friendships, relationships, and extracurricular activities. Very often, anxiety around independence will increase during the transition into college, when a teenager is required to be the most independent they have ever been.

While your teenager might not verbalize the importance of their own independence, they are often looking at you for reassurance. Teenagers feel relieved knowing their parents have confidence in their ability to be independent. When parents continuously intrude or force themself into their teenager's therapy, it sends destructive messages that can increase anxiety. While these messages are often interpreted on a subconscious level, teenagers can feel when their parents do not believe or trust their abilities. This can be scary and very detrimental to a teenager's sense of self and self-esteem.

When a parent provides healthy space, freedom, and independence in therapy, the teenager believes in their own success. The teenager can feel confident in their ability to complete tasks, gain a better sense of self, and feel less anxious. This is a subtle yet strong way for you to support your teenager in coping with anxiety. Additionally, therapy is the perfect place to allow your teenager to have independence. Your teenager is under the care of a professional specialized in this area.

Independence Through Individual Therapy

"My parents are always asking me what I'm talking about during therapy and what I've learned. I'm starting to get anxious about coming to therapy because I know they will press me for information."

–14-YEAR-OLD CLIENT

In continuing to foster independence, refrain from making your teenager's therapist your individual therapist or the designated family therapist. This can be difficult if there are larger familial issues, such as divorce, death, or other concerns with parents or siblings. If this is the case, seek a separate therapist for ongoing family therapy.

Overall, remember the heightened importance of independence during adolescence. Your teenager's therapy sessions might be the only place where they have space and privacy. Many teenagers feel more comfortable sharing information with their therapist, knowing no other family members will be involved. I am often met with the most resistance from teenage clients when there is a fear of a parent "finding out" the content of the therapy sessions, or when a parent insists on joining sessions. Most teenagers enjoy knowing the therapist is "their" therapist and has little connection to people in their personal lives.

Fostering independence also includes refraining from family sessions to discuss what your teenager has learned in therapy. Parents are typically coming from a thoughtful place in this request, but a teenager does not want therapy to become a classroom. Comparing therapy with school, a setting of academic and social stress can be disastrous. While teenagers are learning tools and techniques in therapy, they do not appreciate being quizzed by their parents. This can cause additional stress, create resentment toward parents, and lead a teenager to reconsider attending therapy.

Offering Support

In understanding the importance of fostering independence, you might still be unsure how to move forward. Your teenager is still a minor, and you are understandably worried about their mental health. It is appropriate to *offer* but not force support to your teenager. For example, express your willingness to schedule a family session if your teenager desires. Or you can ask your teenager if they would like you to join their individual session sometime. This allows your teenager to feel your support while respecting their independence. Moreover, many of my clients show more receptivity towards family check-ins when it is scheduled on their terms.

I will note that seeking *occasional* insight or advice from your teenager's therapist is fine. A check-in session with your teenager from time to time can also be appropriate, as long as it is not forced or to discuss what tools they have learned, like a school quiz. In my own practice, I encourage a check-in session with parents, but only if my client is willing. This is something we will discuss at length in the next step, but for now, consider how often you contact your teenager's therapist or insist on check- in sessions. With this being said, if there is an emergency, contact your teenager's therapist right away.

If your teenager has been self-harming, using drugs, or threatening to hurt themselves or others, call their therapist.

Step 3: Be a Guest Star

In continuing to foster independence, "Be a Guest Star" in your teenager's therapy. This third step, "Be a Guest Star" will be particularly helpful if Step 2 was challenging to grasp. Envision the television show scenario to better understand this imperative step.

Television Show Scenario

Imagine your teenager's therapy as a television show that airs once a week for one hour. Your teenager stars as the main character of the show, and the plot centers around their life. The topics of this show might include the main character's friendships, relationships, sexuality, academics, and family dynamics. At this point, the show might start to sound more like a drama than a sitcom! Now, envision yourself as a *guest star* who appears on this television show occasionally.

I receive mixed reactions from parents when I encourage them to envision themselves as guest stars in their teenager's therapy. This is common, as it can evoke feelings of frustration, pain, and even sadness in parents. At one point, you were the main character in your child's life. Prior to adolescence, your child might have looked only to you for guidance and wanted to include you in everything. Now, being regarded as a "guest star," rather than a main character, can make you feel unimportant or pushed to the side. However, you are still a pivotal character in your teenager's life, whether your teenager admits it or not.

Despite understanding this concept, it can still be difficult to let go of your role as a main character in your teenager's therapy. You might not like the idea of your teenager being the only main character in therapy, and you want to be a weekly regular on the show. Maybe you would even like to be a main character again. So, why wouldn't you make yourself a regular weekly character in your teenager's therapy, or even on the same level as the main character? Particularly if your teenager is speaking with their therapist about you or other members of your family in therapy?

This is your teenager's time to be the main character of the show. In fact, your teenager might feel that therapy is the *only* time where they are allowed, and even encouraged, to be the main character of the show. Honoring this concept shows your teenager that you respect their privacy and independence. Furthermore, this can lessen your teenager's anxiety, increase their self-worth, and enhance their relationship with you.

How to Be a Guest Star That Gets Welcomed Back

In considering your new role as a guest star in your teenager's therapy, you may now be asking yourself some of the following questions:

- "What does it mean to be a guest star?"
- "What does it look like to be a guest star?"
- "What if there are serious family issues occurring and it's too risky to be a guest star?"
- "What if I need my time to be a main character?"

Remember, you are still a character on the show. Your character will be welcomed back when you continue to *offer*, but not *force* yourself onto the show.

Translating this analogy from a television show to therapy can appear as:

- Encouraging occasional check-in sessions with your teenager.
- Offering to attend individual sessions.

- Respecting your teenager's privacy by not constantly contacting your teenager's therapist for information (unless in an emergency).

- Remembering this is your teenager's time and not yours.

When Being a Guest Star is Not Enough

You might not have issues respecting your teenager's individual therapy, but still feel more support is needed. You offer to attend therapy with your teenager and maybe schedule a check-in session from time to time. You are handling everything beautifully and respectfully. However, what if there are larger familial issues occurring that extend outside of individual therapy? What if you feel individual therapy is not enough and familial involvement is necessary? Being a guest star who is welcomed back can be tricky when ongoing family therapy is required.

This can be a difficult path to navigate, so engage in an honest conversation with your teenager. Ask their thoughts on attending family therapy and selecting a family therapist. Do not force ongoing family therapy with your teenager's therapist without having a two-sided conversation. Most teenagers hate the idea of sharing their individual therapist with the rest of their family. However, some teens are comfortable using their therapist for both individual therapy, as well as ongoing family therapy. Honor your teenager's decision and respect their feelings.

Furthermore, consider scheduling family therapy in addition to individual therapy, not as a replacement. Many of my clients expressed anger when they were pushed into family therapy instead of individual therapy. This is the complete opposite of a parent acting as a guest star. This action can feel as if a parent canceled the show without permission and replaced it with one where the teenager is no longer the main character. If possible, remind your teenager that they can continue individual therapy while also attending family therapy. In having this conversation, you are again acknowledging and valuing your teenager's input. This is another simple and effective technique to heighten your teenager's self-esteem and lessen anxiety.

If your teenager continues with both individual therapy and family therapy with a separate therapist, be sure to inform the individual therapist. If desired, you and your teenager can complete a Release of Information form (ROI) for the individual therapist to communicate with the family therapist outside of sessions. An ROI allows the individual therapist to collaborate with the family therapist when needed. This is a professional and legal way for two therapists to work together to better help their clients.

Speak with your teenager about the ROI before you decide to sign anything on their behalf. Even though teenagers are minors, it is still important to value their opinion on the matter. Some teenagers might be opposed, but many of my own clients appreciate it when I relay certain information to their family therapist. This can assist clients in meeting their goals while keeping their parents as guest stars.

Case Study

16-year-old "Johnny" came to therapy for anxiety and depression. Johnny's father had cheated on his mother and recently moved out of state. Johnny's parents were in the process of getting a divorce, and Johnny was living full-time with his mother.

Johnny felt immense depression and anxiety surrounding the change in his family. He struggled to attend school and participate in social events. While Johnny often attempted to communicate his feelings to his mother, he did so in a manner that seemed angry and rude. Johnny's mother did not know how to help Johnny. She wanted to respect his individual therapy, but knew he was struggling.

Fortunately, Johnny and his mother began working with a separate family therapist. Johnny and his mother were open to signing a release of information, so I could communicate with the family therapist. The family therapist and I brainstormed ways to help Johnny and his mother. I suggested the family therapist bring up Johnny's feelings surrounding the divorce during family therapy and provide me with feedback after the session. In the meantime, I worked individually with Johnny on how to improve his communication skills.

Through the collaboration of family and individual therapy, Johnny's anxiety and depression lessened. Johnny felt validated and listened to by his mother, and Johnny's mother noticed his improvement in communication. Johnny also appreciated his mother allowing independence during individual therapy and addressing familial matters with the family therapist.

A Final Note on Guest Stardom

Becoming comfortable with being a guest in your teenager's therapy can require patience. Guest stardom might motivate you to pursue additional family therapy with your teenager or perhaps inspire you to seek personal therapy. Your own individual therapy can be a wonderful way to become a separate main character from your teenager. Individual therapy for yourself is particularly beneficial if you are struggling with the idea of being a guest star and feel resistant to Step 3.

Step 4: Respect Privacy Outside of Therapy

Respecting privacy outside of therapy might sound like an easy step, but many parents forget its importance. Parents mean well, but diminish the significance of privacy outside of sessions. It is the 21st century, and views surrounding mental health have changed drastically. People are more open about therapy, and the stigma has lessened. Many people feel comfortable sharing with their waiter at lunch they just came from a therapy session, or talking to their friends at the gym about searching for a therapist. Therefore, you might ask yourself, who *isn't* in therapy?

While I personally love openness surrounding therapy and mental health, keep your teenager's therapy private. Unless your teenager permits you to tell others about their therapy, respect their privacy. With this being said, do not keep this private in a shaming or secretive manner, or because therapy is embarrassing. Rather, respect privacy in a way which honors your teenager's independence. Many teenagers are very open about mental health and may not have a problem with you sharing this information. However, ask your teenager before you share with anyone, even your best friend or your teenager's siblings.

Be mindful of your teen's privacy throughout the entirety of the therapeutic process. Many parents are understanding of this step at first, but as time goes on, they can forget the significance of respecting privacy. If your teenager gives you permission to share that they are in therapy, I still recommend checking in from time to time.

You can ask questions such as:

- "Are you still comfortable with me sharing that you are in therapy?"
- "Who do you feel comfortable with knowing this information?"
- "What are some situations in which you definitely would not want this information shared?"

Respecting privacy and independence continues to show your teenager they are able to trust and confide in you. Thus, you become even more of a support figure they can lean on during times of stress and hardship. Establishing trust in their parents is another wonderful way for teenagers to feel safe and comfortable. As a reminder, feelings of safety and comfort are crucial in combating feelings of worry and anxiety.

Lastly, respecting privacy outside of therapy can lessen your teenager's fear that the world knows about their anxiety. Several of my teenage clients expressed anger towards their parents upon learning they shared about their teenagers' therapy without permission. If you are unsure, and have not yet had this discussion, do not share that your child is in therapy. Overall, do not disclose details about your teenager's therapy to your book club, co-workers, the person you sit next to on a plane, and so forth, unless approved by your teenager.

CHAPTER 11

Tools for Support

The following chapter provides three final steps regarding your teenager receiving additional support. Ensure you are comfortable with Steps 1–4 prior to moving onto Step 5.

Step 5: Discuss Before Recommending

As you continue to respect your teenager's independence, both in and outside of therapy, you can now apply these principles to Step 5: Discuss Before Recommending. This step is fairly similar to Step 4, as it is also frequently forgotten as time goes on. In order to gain a better understanding of the importance of Step 5, once again envision yourself as a teenager.

Teenage Therapy Exercise: Visualization

Imagine yourself as a teenager in therapy. Feel the freedom and relief in speaking with a professional who is unbiased and has your best interests at heart. Envision your parents respecting your safe therapy space. Your parents are no longer calling your therapist, insisting on attending your sessions, or seeking to know what you have learned during therapy. Instead, your parents value privacy and perhaps are now working with their own, separate therapist. Your parents also address familial issues to the family therapist, rather than intruding on your individual sessions. Feel yourself at peace in this situation.

Now, picture yourself coming to therapy and seeing other teenagers you know in the waiting room. You feel completely caught off guard and had no idea your therapist treated your peers. Some of these teenagers could be your mother's friend's kids or perhaps your dad's co-worker's children. You might attend school with these peers and spend many hours of the day together. Perhaps you have socialized with these people or even dated them. When you ask your peers why they are in the waiting room, they reply, "Your parents gave my parents the number for this therapist! I heard this therapist helped you so much!" You are completely surprised and caught off guard. You had no idea your parents recommended your therapist to other people.

What's The Big Deal?

How would you have felt as a teenager in this situation?

While there is no right or wrong answer to this question, I have received a variety of responses from parents. Some parents describe that they would feel uncomfortable in this particular situation and would not like seeing people they know in the waiting room. However, other parents would have no issues working with the same therapist as other people in their immediate life. I have found this to be a common response for parents who are either very open about mental health or live in a small community.

In many communities, particularly small sized communities, some situations cannot be avoided and these types of run-ins are fairly common. Many adults are used to visiting the same dentist, chiropractor or general doctor as their friends, and most likely see the same therapist. Therefore, many of these adults might ask, why would there be a difference in the teenage therapy world? What is the harm in recommending your teenager's therapist to your friend's children without permission from the teenager?

Some of you may also be thinking; "My teenager will never know I recommended my best friend's kid to the same therapist."

I will also note, therapists are bound by confidentiality and can never provide information about their clients to each other. In my practice, I do not share where my referrals come from and how clients originally contacted me to begin therapy. I also do my best to prevent my clients from running into each other in the waiting room or other shared office spaces. However, I cannot truly control whom my clients see outside of the session or determine what my clients say to other clients. Therefore, engage in an open conversation with your teenager surrounding any recommendations.

Open Conversations

> "I just found out my mom told all her friends about me coming here for therapy. Now all my mom's friends want to send their kids here to see you. I would be mortified if I saw them in the waiting room. I'm so upset with my mom."
>
> —14-YEAR-OLD CLIENT

In addition to respecting privacy and independence, it is essential for teenagers to feel they have a say in their therapeutic experience. In the past, several of my teenage clients expressed discomfort after running into someone they knew in the waiting room, only to learn their parents recommended them without permission. A few of these clients expressed the desire to maintain complete separation between the outside world and their therapeutic space. Other clients did not mind seeing their friends in the waiting room, and were happy these people were receiving support. However, each one of these clients described frustration toward their parents for not asking prior to recommending them.

To avoid any increased anxiety, frustration, or discomfort, speak with your teenager before providing any recommendations. Recommendations apply to family, friends, and colleagues. Even if you believe that your teenager will never learn about your recommendations, there is a chance they might. Teenagers can be very private, and seeing someone they know in the context of therapy can be damaging. There is potential for increased anxiety, a desire to switch therapists, beginning the therapist search again, or terminating therapy.

Engaging in an honest conversation eliminates unnecessary stress and helps your teenager feel included in the therapeutic process. As always, facilitate this conversation in a non-forceful and gentle manner, and respect your teenager's final decision. Even as adults, we appreciate it when people ask for our input and respect our feelings.

Step 6: Lessen Pressure

"Pressure is the source of my anxiety. I know it's part of life, but pressure feeds my fears

> in unhealthy ways. I wish there were some pressures that could just go away."
>
> —16-YEAR-OLD CLIENT

You are on a fantastic path in supporting your teenager by completing these first five steps. You are fostering independence, respecting decisions, and engaging in open-ended conversations. Now, lessen any form of pressure for your teenager to be "cured."

"Are You Done Yet?"

It might not have been a strenuous process for your teenager to participate in therapy. Even if your teenager was open to starting therapy, and if finding a therapist was their idea, it is crucial that your teenager does not feel pressured to be "complete" in their emotional growth.

Many of my clients have expressed animosity towards their parents and exhibited anxiety regarding the following situations:

- To be "fixed" or "done" with therapy in a certain timeline or by a specific date.
- To be frequently asked if they need to keep attending therapy.

- To be questioned on how they are meeting their goals and what exactly they are accomplishing in therapy.

- To be reminded about the expense and financial burden of therapy.

These are not unusual questions, as most parents simply want to help their teenager as soon as possible. Who wants to wait for gradual change with anything, especially in regard to their children?

Change requires patience, and it is important to honor your teenager's process. Consider how you feel when placed under pressure to change emotionally, particularly by a specific date. How do you feel when someone wants to know exactly how you are changing and requests a detailed account of the process? You might even be stressed or annoyed just thinking about this situation. Much like you, it is common for teenagers to also feel negatively about pressure.

Turning Down the Pressure Cooker

Consider the additional pressures your teenager already experiences. These might include academic deadlines, advanced placement exams, and college applications. Your teenager could also be dealing with social pressures discussed in Chapter 3. Additionally, your teenager most likely has teachers, tutors, academic counselors, as well as extracurricular coaches checking work, correcting mistakes, and managing their activities.

While this is often required for certain educational and extracurricular endeavors, acknowledge that your teenager lives in an adolescent pressure cooker. Teenagers with anxiety might be reaching a limit on the pressure cooker, or have already gone over their limit. In my own practice, I have seen the limit reached when teenagers feel their parents are micromanaging or pressuring their therapeutic process. This is another reason why I advise monitoring how often you ask your teenager what they are accomplishing in therapy, and if they are done with therapy yet. In fact, you can be a crucial support by *turning down* the pressure cooker, rather than turning the pressure cooker up. If possible, inform your teenager that they do not have a deadline to complete therapy.

Checking In *Without* Pressure

While turning down the pressure cooker, you can still check in with your teenager about their feelings surrounding therapy. It is appropriate to check in from time to time, rather than ignoring the fact that your teenager is in therapy. However, be mindful of the amount you check in. If you are in doubt, practice compassion, and remember your teenager lives in a pressure cooker with a variety of stress factors.

To keep the pressure cooker low, *occasionally* check in with your teenager about the process of therapy in a non-intrusive manner. Once again, facilitate a non-forceful conversation without demands. If your teenager is receptive to the conversation, ask open-ended questions about their feelings surrounding therapy. Avoid mentioning deadlines or pressuring your teenager to finish therapy. Pressuring and placing timelines on a teenager can create annoyance, anxiety, and can also indirectly send the message they are "broken" and "need to be fixed."

As a reminder, the message of "being broken," is very destructive for a teenager's self-esteem. How would you feel if you were told something was wrong with you? Even as an adult, this most likely would not feel positive. To refrain from sending this message, do not pressure your teenager to complete therapy. Instead, focus on feelings surrounding therapy, and as always, applaud your teenager for using therapy as a resource.

If your teenager is not willing to engage in a check-in conversation, respect their privacy and move on. Forcing or insisting on a conversation turns up the pressure cooker and ultimately pushes your teenager farther away. Your own individual therapy is a fantastic way to find additional support in this area.

Examine Your Own Pressure Cooker

Prior to moving on to Step 7, reflect on your own personal pressure cooker level. Many parents understand the importance of lessening pressure on their teenagers in regard to the process of therapy. However, there can be situational factors that can lead parents to turn up the pressure cooker without realizing it. I have found this to be common when there are financial constraints, or if therapy was not something originally desired.

The Money Pressure Cooker

> "I really want my kid to keep attending therapy. I just can't afford it and it's causing anxiety within me. I feel so lost. I don't know what to do."
>
> —Parent of 14-year-old client

If your finances are limited, it can be challenging not to pressure your teenager about deadlines surrounding therapy. If money is tight, and there are few funds you can use towards therapy, what are you supposed to do? You have bills to pay and food to put on the table for your family. Long-term therapy might not be an option, even if you and your teenager would like it to be. This is a very difficult situation, particularly when you want to support your teenager.

If there are financial reasons as to why your teenager needs to stop therapy, speak with your teenager's therapist. It is entirely appropriate to ask your teenager's therapist if they can reduce their rate or offer a sliding scale fee. As mentioned earlier, therapists possess different policies surrounding sliding scale fees and might have the flexibility to reduce their rate on a temporary or long-term basis. If your teenager's therapist cannot offer a lower fee, respect the decision, and begin to search for a new therapist.

As discussed in Chapter 9, there are many mental health resources offering therapy at a low-cost or on a sliding scale. You can search for non-profit groups or centers where therapy is provided by trainees under supervision. Although it is not ideal for your teenager to switch therapists too often, if support is still needed, do your best to find a new therapist.

Even if you are overly stressed with the finances of therapy, try not to over-share with your teenager. Avoid bombarding your teenager with complaints about the expense of therapy, and how miserable it is to pay their therapy bills. I have seen this often in my practice, and many times from caring parents who do not realize the effect this has on their teenager. Complaints can create guilt, stress, and additional anxiety for teenagers about receiving support. Once again, these statements also indirectly send a message that the teenager is "problematic" and "an inconvenience."

Although it is valid to feel the stress of financial hardship, let out your feelings in healthy ways that do not directly involve your teenager. Write in your journal, meditate, exercise, and practice your own coping skills. While I advise not oversharing the financial burden of therapy, inform your teenager that therapy is a serious commitment. It is crucial for teenagers to be aware that they need to attend their appointments on time and not to cancel unless it is a true emergency.

The Therapy-Reluctant Pressure Cooker

A parent's pressure cooker can also heighten when there are conflicting feelings about therapy. As explored in Chapter 10, it is helpful to have both parents support their teenager's therapeutic process. However, what if your partner, or your teenager's other parent, did not want your teenager to attend therapy in the first place? Or, what if you were the parent that did not understand the point of therapy, but reluctantly agreed? If your partner, teenager's other parent, or even you, do not truly understand the point of therapy, you might find yourself wanting to place a limit on your teenager's therapeutic process. You could also be tired of hearing your partner's complaints about therapy or have lost patience in waiting for slow improvement in your teenager.

If this feels relatable, remember this process is about your teenager, and not about you, your partner, or your teenager's other parent. Even if your partner or teenager's other parent does not believe therapy would work for them, therapy can still benefit your teenager. Similarly, it is okay if therapy is not your cup of tea. However, keep your feelings about therapy and its timeline separate from your teenager. Allow your teenager to have space and freedom in therapy and take their time in their journey of self-discovery. Let therapy be a refuge away from completion deadlines, pressure, or stress.

Case Study

16-year-old client "Tony" was referred to therapy by his high school counselor. In our first meeting, Tony described feeling unsure about seeking therapy for support. Tony explained his mother was supportive of therapy and wanted him to visit a therapist for the past several years. Tony noted his father was highly opposed to therapy, stating it was a waste of time and money.

Tony explained how this dynamic was not uncommon among his parents. Tony's parents disagreed on many subjects, and did not hide this from Tony. In addition to experiencing anxiety around school and social dynamics, Tony confessed he now also felt anxious about therapy. Tony feared he was disappointing his father by attending therapy but knew he needed support and trusted his mother. This dilemma added to Tony's already existing anxiety.

Thankfully, Tony and his parents were receptive to a check-in session in which we could discuss this issue. Tony's father remained grounded in his beliefs about therapy, and felt therapy would not work for him. However, Tony's father was open to no longer sharing these thoughts with his son. Instead, Tony's father acknowledged that Tony might benefit from therapeutic support. By respecting Tony's choice to pursue therapy, Tony and I could focus on alleviating his academic and social anxieties.

TOOLS FOR SUPPORT

Step 7: Therapy as a Continued Resource

"It helps me feel less anxious just knowing I have support through therapy. I feel safer knowing I can reach out when I'm struggling."

—17-YEAR-OLD CLIENT

The final step in supporting your teenager's therapeutic process is fairly simple: allow your teenager to use therapy as a continued resource. There will come a time when your teenager begins to notice positive changes. Anxiety lessens, self-esteem increases, and your teenager expresses the desire to stop therapy. Your teenager and their therapist mutually decide to either terminate therapeutic services or pause regular, ongoing sessions. This is an exciting time, as it typically indicates that your teenager has reached their goals.

When this time comes, inform your teenager that they can return to therapy in the future. Life has unexpected twists and turns, and new concerns can arise as your teen moves forward. Share with your teenager that there is no requirement to be perfect and "fixed" now that they have decided to stop therapy. If your teenager would like to return to therapy in the future, do your best to support their decision. Provide options as to whether your teenager would like to return to the original therapist or find a new provider. It can be an incredible relief for your teenager to learn they have this resource available. Additionally, your approval and support can make the return to therapy more comfortable.

Continued Therapy with Goal Completion

Therapy as a continued resource also applies prior to your teenager terminating therapeutic services.

Parents of clients in my private practice frequently ask the following questions:

- "Is it okay for my teenager to continue therapy, even after their anxiety decreases and they meet their goals?"

- "My teenager would like to keep working with their therapist but my teenager seems better. Is this helpful or unhelpful?"

- "Is it constructive to schedule check-in sessions once per month? Or better to terminate therapy?"

It can be confusing how to proceed once your teenager has shown improvements and is beginning to meet their goals. When someone visits a doctor to treat an infection, they typically do not return to the doctor once the infection is healed. Therefore, you might question, does therapy work the same way?

Since all individuals are different, there are a variety of ways to use therapy as a continued resource. Some teenagers feel they are ready to stop therapy once they reach their initial goals. With their parents' support, these teenagers can return to therapy in the future and will reach out to their therapist if need be. However, other teenagers benefit from continuing to meet with their therapist on a regular basis. As a therapist, I believe there is absolutely nothing wrong with this. Leaning on a consistent support figure outside of one's immediate, day-to-day life can feel calming and relieving.

Maintenance Therapy

"Maintenance therapy" is when a teenager continues therapy after reaching their initial goals. During maintenance therapy, there might not be an immediate crisis, but smaller concerns arise which benefit from support. I personally feel that maintenance therapy can be equally as powerful as therapy during the beginning of treatment. Several of my clients report that maintenance therapy prevented anxiety from reoccurring at the same level of intensity as when they first sought therapy. Maintenance therapy provides a consistent resource for teenagers, while providing space to process experiences, both minor and major.

Furthermore, maintenance therapy is a fantastic way for teenagers to delve into any deeper, underlying issues that could have originally influenced their anxiety. In most scenarios, teenagers begin working with a therapist to stop anxiety as soon as possible. In this initial phase of therapy, the teenager begins to establish rapport with their therapist and learns new coping skills, emotional regulation techniques, and stress management tools. This helps manage anxiety and prevent anxiety from increasing in the future. While this is highly important, the initial phase of therapy might not allow for the processing of what's occurring underneath the surface.

Maintenance therapy is when a teenager can fully explore what's going on "underneath the surface," after the initial crisis is resolved. Maintenance therapy allows flexibility to discuss topics such as childhood experiences, sense of self, identity, relationships, and future goals that can contribute to anxiety on a more subconscious level. During maintenance therapy, the majority of the time is no longer spent discussing specific coping skills, but instead focuses on healing the *root* of anxiety.

Another significant aspect of maintenance therapy is increased comfort and familiarity with the therapist. Many teenagers struggle to address the underlying cause of anxiety at the onset of therapy. It takes time to feel comfortable with a new therapist, and it can be scary to delve into underlying issues without a trusting bond. Typically, when a teenager reaches the point of maintenance therapy, they have established a safe and secure connection with their therapist. Thus, maintenance therapy can be a time of immense vulnerability and healing for teenagers.

In addition to processing underlying concerns, maintenance therapy can also prompt teenagers to set new and revised goals. As adults, we are constantly growing and evolving, so why would teenagers be any different? It is healthy and constructive for teenagers to set new aspirations as they mature into adulthood. Maintenance therapy can create new goals that are related, but not solely focused on the elimination of anxiety. In my own practice, I have found the goals set during maintenance therapy to be beneficial for a teenager's present and future.

Case Study

17-year-old "Giselle" came to therapy at the start of her senior year of high school. While Giselle thrived socially, she struggled in school, and academics were highly stress-inducing. Giselle's anxiety was so severe that she would often throw up before tests and presentations.

Giselle and I worked on immediate coping skills and ways for Giselle to self-regulate. Giselle was an excellent therapy client as she practiced these tools daily, even when she didn't feel anxious. When Giselle was faced with a big test or presentation, she would lean on her coping skills and was able to persevere. Giselle was thrilled she had met her initial therapy goals; her anxiety lessened, and her confidence increased.

While Giselle had accomplished her goals, she expressed the desire to remain in therapy. Since Giselle's initial crisis had subsided, we were able to use maintenance therapy to explore underlying factors contributing to anxiety. We examined Giselle's sense of self and self-esteem, and processed early childhood experiences.

The combination of crisis management and maintenance therapy helped Giselle feel more prepared for life after high school. Giselle noted she would not have attended college away from home if it were not for maintenance therapy. At the current time, Giselle is a junior in college and continues to reach out for check-in sessions as needed.

Maintenance Therapy as a Supplement

If you are unsure about maintenance therapy, consider this analogy: Imagine maintenance therapy as the mental health version of vitamin supplements. If you know your immune system is compromised, you might take vitamins on a regular basis to boost your strength and prevent illness. Over time, you might notice your immune system growing stronger from consistency with your vitamin routine. This is similar to the process of maintenance therapy. Maintenance therapy works on a covert or subtle level, but in the long term, it is very helpful. Maintenance therapy can manage your teenager's anxiety while addressing underlying issues, and can be a resource during times of unexpected stress.

While some parents might be opposed to the idea of maintenance therapy, it is important to once again remember this is your teenager's journey. Engage in a conversation with your teenager about their thoughts on maintenance therapy. If your teenager wants to continue with therapy, practice compassion and empathy in allowing this to be an option. Maintenance therapy can also include modifying therapy meetings to a biweekly or monthly basis. Most importantly, discuss all options with your teenager, and ensure both your teenager and their therapist feel comfortable with the final decision.

A Consistent, Continued Resource

> "I really like that my parents are cool about me reaching out for additional therapy sessions when I'm stressed or going through something. I'm lucky my parents are like that."
>
> —14-YEAR-OLD CLIENT

Lastly, use therapy as a consistent and continued resource, regardless of the therapy timeline. This applies to teenagers who are new to therapy, consistent with sessions, in a maintenance phase, or have terminated therapy. If your teenager is struggling at any point, suggest scheduling an additional therapy session. However, it is essential to offer this option, rather than force your teenager to contact their therapist. Remind your teenager that additional therapy is an option during times of hardship. Not only does this action show support and understanding, but it also validates your teenager's desire for guidance and assistance. This portrays your acceptance of their process, as well as the value of practicing self-care.

I will also note, that therapists possess different protocols surrounding additional sessions. In my practice, I try to keep at least one opening a day for when a client is struggling and would like an extra session. As a parent, you can encourage your teenager to speak with their therapist about the policies on extra sessions. Some therapists might also offer longer or "double" sessions, which typically range around 90 minutes, rather than the standard 45 or 60 minutes. These can be useful options when more sessions are temporarily needed.

If your teenager continues to struggle, it can be beneficial to schedule ongoing therapy more than once a week. This can be advantageous on a long- or short-term basis, depending on the teenager and the specific situation. Again, speak with your teenager and their therapist prior to making any decisions. If your teenager and their therapist request more sessions, express support, non-judgement, and understanding.

CHAPTER 12

Additional Holistic Resources

In addition to the resources related to traditional psychotherapy, consider holistic adjunct forms of healing. These modalities are not to replace the resources delegated to treating anxiety, but can be valuable supplements. Many mental health treatment centers frequently incorporate these services alongside individual psychotherapy and psychiatry.

Some alternate and adjunct treatment modalities for alleviating anxiety might include:

- Group therapy
- 12-step recovery
- Massage
- Acupuncture
- Acupressure
- Reiki and other forms of energy healing
- Reflexology

- Chiropractic
- Yoga
- Meditation
- Breathwork
- Spiritual learning and development
- Sound healing
- Team sports and athletics
- Dance and movement
- Exercise (boxing, lifting weights, swimming)
- Martial arts
- Art
- Music
- Design
- Creative writing
- Journaling
- Nutritional coaching
- Animal-assisted therapy
- Art therapy
- Drama therapy
- Movement therapy
- Music therapy
- Horticultural therapy

Overall, seek supplemental holistic resources that work for your teenager. Ask your teenager what sparks their curiosity, and if they are open to exploring. With this being said, do not force your teenager or overload their schedule with activities. If your teenager specifically says no, honor their choice and, if appropriate, return to the conversation in the future.

Encourage your teenager to engage in at least one activity a week that nourishes self-care. This might be an activity or

ADDITIONAL HOLISTIC RESOURCES

resource from the list above, or an activity I have not mentioned. You could also ask your teenager if they would like you to join the activity the first time, or if they prefer privacy. However, I only recommend this option if your teenager is enthusiastic about the concept of a shared activity.

Remember, what works for you might not appeal to your teenager. You might love yoga and meditation, whereas your teenager prefers martial arts or lifting weights at the gym. Gently encourage your teenager, rather than forcing them to engage in an activity of your choosing. Speak with your teenager about what feels right and listen to their decision.

Conclusion

There is a plethora of information provided throughout this book, so take your time to digest the topics. Most importantly, credit yourself for your willingness and openness in reading the material and engaging in your own self-reflection. This is often a daunting and challenging task, and it is crucial that you do not overlook your own strength.

Remember, you and your teenager are on a journey of growth. It is imperative to practice compassion and empathy, and to understand there is not an immediate cure for anxiety. It can take time to to notice change and adjustments in your teen's anxiety levels. Calming anxiety is not an overnight process, so patience will be your best friend throughout this process.

Lastly, do not be limited by simply reading this book. I do not have all the answers, and I advise researching and absorbing as much information as possible. Your knowledge is power, and the more you learn, the better resource you can be for your teenager. As a reminder, this book is not intended to substitute any type of professional help. Join support groups, work with an individual and/or family therapist, learn from different teachers, and read a variety of books about teenage mental health. The more open you are to learning, the better.

As a therapist, I am truly grateful for parents like you. You have made tremendous strides in reading this book and are helping to heal those around you. I wish you well on your journey in guiding and supporting your teenager with anxiety. Please feel free to visit my website www.sophiagalano.com with any questions or comments.

Acknowledgements

My deepest gratitude goes to everyone who helped make this book a reality and bring it to life.

Thank you to everyone at Hatherleigh Press, and to Hilda Brucker for encouraging me to pursue a traditional publisher. To Kathe Crawford for being so positive and enthusiastic about my writing. Thank you to Martha Koo, my mentor and friend for almost ten years. Thank you to Phil Zuckerman for inspiring me since your first class my freshman year. To Sheril Antonio, for the support and writing such lovely praise. Thank you to Jaime Ryan for the constant laughs while working in a truly difficult field. To Brittany Plut, for your enthusiasm and calming presence.

Thank you to Annie for always being by my side, and bringing such good into my life since the day I met you. Thank you to my parents for always encouraging me to be independent and grow into my own. Laurette, for always being there and supporting every single one of my creative endeavors. Julian, for the PR guidance and more laughs. Thank you to Robert; you are amazing and help so many people.

Last but certainly not least, thank you to my amazing husband, Mitch Jackson. My rock through everything and my biggest supporter.

About the Author

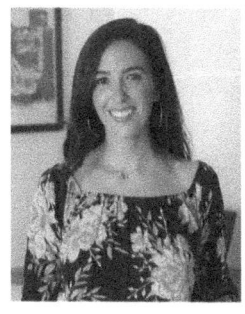

Sophia Vale Galano was born in Los Angeles, raised in London, and holds a Master's degree in Social Work from New York University. Sophia earned her LCSW in 2018 and has a thriving therapy practice, catering to adults and teenagers throughout California. Additionally, Sophia has extensive experience working as a therapist in residential, inpatient, outpatient, medical, and educational settings, for both adolescents and adults. In conjunction with running a private practice, Sophia supervises associate therapists.

In addition to her work as a therapist, Sophia is a certified yoga instructor, Master Reiki Practitioner, and volunteers for several nonprofit organizations. After achieving her LCSW, Sophia completed a Sex Therapy certification from California Institute of Integral Studies, an Animal Assisted Therapy certification from The Animal Behavior Institute, and a Forensic Social Work Certification from The National Organization of Forensic Social Work.